POST-TRAUMATIC STRESS DISORDER and CHRONIC HEALTH CONDITIONS

Edited by Steven S. Coughlin, PhD

D1496792

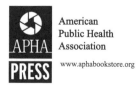

American Public Health Association

APHA

PRESS

www.aphabookstore.org

WASHINGTON, D.C. ● 2012

American Public Health Association
800 I Street, NW
Washington, DC 20001-3710
www.apha.org

Georges C. Benjamin, MD, FACP, FACEP (Emeritus), Executive Director
Anne B. Keith, RN, DrPH, C-PNP, Publications Board Liaison
Judith C. Hays, PhD, RN, Publications Board Liaison

Printed and bound in the United States of America
Production Editor: Teena Lucas
Typesetting: The Charlesworth Group
Cover Design: Alan Giarcanella
Printing and Binding: Victor Graphics Inc., Baltimore, MD

Library of Congress Cataloging-in-Publication Data

Coughlin, Steven S. (Steven Scott), 1957-
Post-traumatic stress disorder and chronic health conditions / by Steven S. Coughlin.
   p. cm.
Includes index.
Includes bibliographical references.
ISBN 978-0-87553-016-1
1. Post-traumatic stress disorder--Complications. 2. Chronic diseases. I. Title.
RC552.P67C67 2012
616.85'21--dc23
                              2011050717

12/2011

TABLE OF CONTENTS

About the Editor

Steven S. Coughlin received his M.P.H. degree from San Diego State University in 1984 and his Ph.D. from The Johns Hopkins University in 1987. Dr. Coughlin lives in the Washington, DC, metropolitan area where he is a member of the Post-Deployment Health Epidemiology Program, Office of Public Health, at the U.S. Department of Veterans Affairs. He is an Adjunct Professor of Epidemiology at the Rollins School of Public Health at Emory University in Atlanta, GA. Previously he was a senior cancer epidemiologist at the Centers for Disease Control and Prevention, in Atlanta, GA, and an Associate Professor of Epidemiology at the Tulane University School of Public Health and Tropical Medicine in New Orleans, LA. Dr. Coughlin is an Associate Editor of the *American Journal of Epidemiology*, Editor-in-Chief of *The Open Health Services and Policy Journal*, a member of the Senior Editorial Board of the *International Journal of Molecular Epidemiology and Genetics*, and a member of the Honorary Editorial Board of *Risk Management and Healthcare Policy*. He is the author or co-author of more than 200 articles and the author or co-editor of several books including *Ethics and Epidemiology* (Oxford University Press, 1996; 2nd edition, 2009), *Case Studies in Public Health Ethics* (American Public Health Association, 1997; 2nd edition, 2009), *The Nature of Principles* (Xlibris, 2008), the second edition of *Ethics in Epidemiology and Public Health Practice: Collected Works* (American Public Health Association, 2009), and *Causal Inference and Scientific Paradigms in Epidemiology* (Bentham Science Publishers, 2010).

Contributors

J. Wesson Ashford, M.D., Ph.D.
Director
War Related Illness and Injury Study Center
Veterans Affairs Palo Alto Health Care System
Clinical Professor (affiliated)
Department of Psychiatry and Behavioral Sciences
Stanford University School of Medicine
Palo Alto, CA

Patrick S. Calhoun, Ph.D.
Clinical Psychologist
Director of Fellowship Training
Durham Veterans Affairs Medical Center and Mid-Atlantic Mental illness
Research, Education, and Clinical Center
Assistant Professor, Department of Psychiatry and Behavioral Sciences
Duke University Medical Center
Durham, NC

Julie C. Chapman, Psy.D.
Director of Neuroscience
Principal Investigator, MIND Study
War Related Illness and Injury Study Center
Veterans Affairs Medical Center
Washington, DC
Assistant Professor of Neurology

Georgetown University School of Medicine
Washington, DC

Steven S. Coughlin, Ph.D., M.P.H.
Senior Epidemiologist
Post-Deployment Health Epidemiology Program
Office of Public Health
Department of Veterans Affairs
Washington, DC
Adjunct Professor of Epidemiology
Rollins School of Public Health
Emory University
Atlanta, GA

Yasmin S. Cypel, Ph.D., M.S.
Post-Deployment Health Epidemiology Program
Office of Public Health
Department of Veterans Affairs
Washington, DC

Laura Herrera, M.D., M.P.H.
Acting Deputy Director
Patient Care Services
Department of Veterans Affairs
Washington, DC

Rebecca Boehm McNeil, Ph.D.
Durham Epidemiologic Research and Information Center
Veterans Affairs Medical Center
Durham, NC

Jennifer Jane Runnals, Ph.D.
Research Psychologist
Veterans Affairs Mid-Atlantic Health Care Network Registry Project
Mental Illness Research, Education, and Clinical Center
Veterans Affairs Medical Center
Durham, NC

Patrick M. Sullivan, M.A.
Research Assistant, Chapman Laboratory
War Related Illness and Injury Study Center
Veterans Affairs Medical Center
Washington, DC

Elizabeth Van Voorhees, Ph.D.
Psychologist
Mental Illness Research, Education, and Clinical Center
Veterans Affairs Medical Center
Assistant Professor
Department of Psychiatry and Behavioral Sciences
Duke University Medical Center
Durham, NC

Preface

Post-traumatic stress disorder (PTSD) is a serious anxiety disorder that can occur among persons exposed to traumatic events. PTSD has been related to several adverse health outcomes and to increased utilization of health care services. The focus of this book is on the relationships between PTSD and chronic health conditions including other psychiatric conditions such as substance abuse and dependency, chronic pain, obesity, diabetes, metabolic syndrome, cardiovascular disease, and traumatic brain injury. Other topics that have not been extensively dealt with in the published literature (for example, the relationships between PTSD and respiratory symptoms and asthma, rheumatoid arthritis, HIV/AIDS, and women's health concerns) are discussed as further examples. Information about comorbidity between PTSD and these chronic conditions includes findings from clinical and epidemiologic studies of military, veteran, and civilian populations as well as neurobiological and behavioral research.

The studies summarized in this book show that there are likely to be multiple pathways by which traumatic events lead to PTSD and other adverse health outcomes. Trauma can lead to several anxiety and mood disorders as well as other psychological conditions, in addition to adverse changes in health risk factors. Although PTSD is unlikely to account for all of the effects of traumatic events on health, it is likely to be a key pathway through which traumatic exposure leads to chronic health outcomes.

The chapters included in Part I of this book provide an overview of PTSD including diagnostic criteria, conceptual issues, family violence and other risk factors for PTSD, as well as biological, genetic, and immunologic mechanisms that are likely to play an important role in the pathogenesis of PTSD and PTSD-related chronic health conditions. The epidemiology of PTSD in civilian, military, and veteran populations is discussed in Chapter 2, including studies of populations exposed to natural and man-made disasters.

In Part II of this book, Chapters 3 and 4 provide an account of the complex relationships between PTSD and other Axis I and Axis II psychiatric disorders including alcohol and drug abuse and dependence. The large body of research summarized in these chapters includes clinical and epidemiologic studies of substance abuse and dependence in civilian and veteran populations. A major focus of the studies summarized in these chapters clarifies the natural history of PTSD and related psychiatric disorders, with the goal of helping to alleviate suffering among persons with comorbid mental health conditions such as PTSD and alcohol dependence.

In Chapter 5, the authors provide an account of the relationships between chronic pain and PTSD. Chronic pain and pain syndromes have long been associated with military service. For example, complex regional pain syndrome, which was previously known as reflex sympathetic dystrophy, was first described during the American Civil War. In recent decades, studies have shown that chronic pain is frequently reported by veterans and that chronic pain is often associated with significant levels of psychological distress and physical disability. Chronic pain and PTSD may interact in such a way that the course of either condition is adversely affected. For example, patients with chronic pain and PTSD may experience more intense pain and affective distress and greater disability than patients with chronic pain without PTSD. A number of factors may account for interactions between chronic pain and PTSD. Pain may be a reminder of the traumatic event and trigger memories of the trauma or avoidance of the cause of pain.

Epidemiological studies of U.S. veterans have shown that pain symptoms and diagnoses are among the most frequent medical conditions among veterans of the 1991 Gulf War and in veterans who served in Operation Enduring Freedom (OEF) and Operation Iraqi Freedom (OIF). Persistent muscle or joint pain and headaches which are not explained by an established, conventional medical or mental disorder diagnosis are among the constellation of symptoms that are frequently reported by Gulf War veterans as part of unexplained multi-symptom illness. Chronic pain is frequently accompanied by impairment of physical function and comorbid psychiatric conditions such as PTSD and depression. A number of factors may account for interactions between chronic pain and PTSD. For example, pain may be a reminder of the traumatic event and trigger memories of the trauma or avoidance of the cause of pain.

Chapters 6 and 7 summarize the burgeoning literature on the relationships between PTSD and obesity, diabetes, metabolic syndrome, and cardiovascular diseases such as coronary heart disease and stroke. In addition to research findings that persons with PTSD are likely to have an increased risk of cardiovascular risk factors and coronary heart disease, an increasing body of evidence indicates that some persons may develop PTSD as a result of suffering a heart attack or other life-threatening illness. As noted in Chapter 7, persons with PTSD have been reported to be more likely to have hypertension, hyperlipidemia, obesity, and cardiovascular disease. However, the causality of some reported associations is unclear from current evidence.

The focus of Chapter 8 is on the co-occurrence of PTSD and traumatic brain injury in civilian, military, and veteran populations including ongoing research aimed at distinguishing between the two conditions among persons exposed to combat-related blast injuries.

The topic of PTSD and chronic health conditions is very large and broadly interconnected with several areas of health, health care services, and public health. The general approach used to identify references cited in the book was to identify relevant medical subject headings (MeSH) used by the National Library of Medicine and to search the National Center for Biotechnology Information PubMed bibliographic databases for appropriate articles. Of particular interest were clinical and epidemiologic studies of PTSD and chronic health conditions published since 1981 when the MeSH heading "Stress disorders, post-traumatic" was first introduced. The bibliographic searches did not focus on studies of psychological or physiological stress published prior to 1981. Clinical descriptions of individual psychiatric patients and case series involving very small numbers of patients were omitted. The bibliographic searches were limited to studies published in English. However, because PTSD and trauma-related health conditions are global health concerns, the bibliographic searches were not limited to studies carried out in the United States. Additional citations were identified by reviewing systematic reviews and review articles identified through PubMed searches (for example, recent review articles on the genetics of PTSD) along with monographs on veterans health topics prepared by the RAND Corporation and the Institute of Medicine. The completeness of the bibliographic database searches was greater for chapters on PTSD in relation to specific chronic health conditions (for example, chronic pain, cardiovascular disease, diabetes, obesity, and traumatic brain injury). In

Chapter 1, where the intent was to provide a broad overview of PTSD, we necessarily omitted some potential citations, because the overall published literature on PTSD and related psychiatric conditions in children, adolescents, and adults is vast.

This book would not have been possible without the support and encouragement of many colleagues who share my enthusiasm for veterans' health research, epidemiology, and psychological research. I am also indebted to anonymous reviewers who were generous with their time and constructive critical comments. Superb assistance was provided by librarians at the Department of Veterans Affairs Central Office. I would especially like to thank Dr. Anne Keith for being our American Public Health Association (APHA) Publications Board liaison and offering several constructive comments for improving the book; Teena Lucas, APHA's Book Production Editor; Nina Tristani, Director of Publications for APHA, and colleagues in the Office of Public Health at the Department of Veterans Affairs in Washington, DC, at the War Related Illness and Injury Study Centers (WRIISC), at the Veterans Affairs (VA) Medical Center in Palo Alto, CA, and in Washington, DC, and at the VA Medical Center in Durham, NC, as well as faculty and students at the Rollins School of Public Health at Emory University in Atlanta, GA. This book is dedicated to the veterans and communities we serve.

Steven S. Coughlin, Ph.D.
Washington, DC

1

Overview of Post-Traumatic Stress Disorder

Steven S. Coughlin, Ph.D., and Rebecca Boehm McNeil, Ph.D.

Post-Traumatic Stress Disorder (PTSD) is an anxiety disorder that can occur after an individual experiences a traumatic event such as a combat experience, a motor vehicle crash, physical assault, or sexual assault. Of course, this list is not exhaustive. People who are robbed, kidnapped, taken hostage, exposed to a terrorist attack, tortured, held as a prisoner of war or in a concentration camp, or exposed to a natural disaster may also respond with intense fear, helplessness, or horror. Symptoms of PTSD develop after exposure to an extreme traumatic stressor involving threatened death, serious injury, or witnessing an event that involves serious injury or death of another person. Symptoms of PTSD may include nightmares, intrusive thoughts, or other reexperiencing phenomena, the avoidance of situations that remind the person of the traumatic event, a feeling of numbness or being socially detached from family and friends, and hyperarousal (for example, feeling angry, irritable and "on edge," or having difficulty concentrating). Hyperarousal or hyper-vigilance includes a rapid and pronounced reaction to stressors which may lead to a preoccupation with signs of threat and emotional distress.

The constellation of (reexperiencing, avoidance, and hyperarousal) symptoms seen with PTSD may be accompanied by impaired modulation of affect, hostility, self-destructive behavior, feelings of ineffectiveness or despair, or a feeling of being permanently damaged in some way (DSM-IV-TR). Persons with PTSD may have other challenges such as difficulties with employment, relationships, or other health conditions (for example, major depression, alcohol abuse, or drug dependency). Studies have shown that male and female veterans with PTSD are less likely to be married, more likely to be divorced, and more likely to have marital problems as compared with veterans without PTSD. The children of veterans with PTSD may experience problems with behavior, school, and relationships, underscoring the value of individual and family therapy as well as a family-oriented approach for alleviating suffering due to PTSD.

The relationship between trauma and PTSD has been the subject of considerable research involving military, veteran, and civilian populations, as discussed throughout this book. Studies in military, veteran, and civilian populations have shown that the risk of developing PTSD increases with the intensity or duration of trauma exposure (Breslau and Davis 1992). In studies of military personnel and veterans, for example, PTSD rates have been shown to rise with increases in the level of combat exposure and number of deployments to combat theatres. A further issue is that trauma can lead to several anxiety and mood disorders and other psychological conditions in addition to PTSD. However, the development of PTSD is likely to be a key pathway through which traumatic exposure leads to adverse health outcomes (Schnurr and Green 2004). Nevertheless, PTSD is unlikely to mediate all of the effect of traumatic events on health (Schnurr and Green 2004). Psychological and biological models of PTSD are summarized below along with a summary of genetic findings in PTSD research. Any complete model of PTSD must account for why many people exposed to extreme stress do not develop PTSD and why some trauma survivors recover and others do not.

DIAGNOSTIC CRITERIA FOR PTSD

According to the Diagnostic and Statistical Manual of Mental Disorders (DSM-IV-TR) the diagnostic criteria for PTSD, is a person who has been exposed to a traumatic event in which both of the following were present: (1) the person experienced, witnessed, or was confronted with an event or events that involved actual or threatened death or serious injury, or a threat to the physical integrity of self or others, and (2) the person's response involved intense fear, helplessness, or horror. These conditions for PTSD are referred to as criterion A. This criterion makes it clear that it is not just the nature of the exposure (e.g., life-threatening heart attack or combat exposures), but also how the person experiences the traumatic event. How the person experiences the traumatic event is influenced by personal factors (e.g., age, gender, prior history of trauma, psychiatric conditions, genetics), social and cultural factors (e.g., lack of social support, stigma, etc.), and factors related to resilience to trauma or extremely stressful events (e.g., positive family relationships, peer support, access to medical care, or positive coping strategies that do not involve substance abuse).

Criterion B requires that the traumatic event is persistently reexperienced in one or more of the following ways: (1) recurrent and intrusive distressing recollections of the event, (2) recurrent distressing dreams of the event, (3) acting or feeling as if the traumatic event were recurring, (4) intense psychological distress at exposure to internal or external cues that resemble an aspect of the traumatic event, and (5) physiological reactivity on exposure to internal or external cues that resemble an aspect of the traumatic event (DSM-IV-TR). Examples of reexperiencing phenomena include a sense of reliving the experience, hallucinations, and brief dissociative episodes sometimes referred to as "flashbacks."

DSM-IV-TR criterion C for PTSD entails the persistent avoidance of stimuli associated with the trauma and numbing of general responsiveness as shown by three or more of the following: (1) efforts to avoid thoughts, feelings, or conversations associated with the trauma, (2) efforts to avoid activities, places, or people that arouse recollections of the trauma, (3) inability to recall an important aspect of the trauma, (4) markedly diminished interest or participation in significant activities, (5) a feeling of detachment or estrange-ment from others, (6) restricted range of affect, and (7) a sense of a fore-shortened future (DSM-IV-TR). Examples of the latter include not expecting to have a career or a normal life span. The person may have a reduced ability to feel emotions such as those associated with intimacy or tenderness.

Criterion D consists of persistent symptoms of increased arousal as shown by two or more of the following: (1) difficulty falling or staying asleep, (2) irritability or outbursts of anger, (3) difficulty concentrating, (4) hypervigilance, and (5) exaggerated startle response. According to DSM-IV-TR criteria E and F, the duration of symptoms must be more than one month, and the symptoms must cause clinically significant distress or impairment in social, occupational, or other important areas of functioning. In the first month following exposure to a traumatic event, people suffering from trauma may meet the criteria for acute stress disorder. PTSD is considered to be acute if the duration is more than one month but less than three months. The duration of chronic PTSD is three months or longer (DSM-IV-TR). If the condition occurs after a delay of 6 months or longer, then it is referred to as delayed onset PTSD.

The DSM-IV-TR criteria recognize that PTSD is likely to be exhibited differently in children than in adults. For example, children may reexperience the traumatic event through repetitive or reenacting play (Margolin and Vickerman 2007).

The next update for DSM (DSM-5) is scheduled for release in 2013 and the American Psychiatric Association has released draft diagnostic criteria for public comment. In these draft diagnostic criteria, criterion A for PTSD (exposure to traumatic events) is more specifically stated, some items in criterion B (intrusion symptoms) are revised, criterion C (avoidance and numbing) is split into two criteria, and there are also revisions in criterion E (formerly D), which focuses on increased arousal.

RISK FACTORS FOR PTSD

Risk factors for PTSD include the severity or duration of exposure to trauma (DSM-IV-TR). PTSD may be especially severe or long lasting when the stressor was of human design (for example, rape or torture). Other risk factors for PTSD include a past history of trauma prior to the index trauma; past history of PTSD, depression or anxiety disorder; and having a positive family history of anxiety or PTSD (Hales et al. 2008). Risk factors that have been identified in epidemiologic studies are further discussed in Chapter 2. Comorbid Axis II disorders are risk factors for a greater chronicity of PTSD, as discussed in Chapter 3. Other risk factors for PTSD include lack of social support from family or friends and disrupted parental attachments (Hales et al. 2008). Risk factors for PTSD that occur early in life are further discussed below in the context of child abuse, neglect, and family violence.

Child Abuse, Neglect, and Family Violence as Risk Factors for PTSD

The literature on PTSD in children, adolescents, and adults intersects with the broad literature on human health and development, because adverse experiences during childhood can have a negative impact on health and well-being throughout the life span. A child's vulnerability to trauma is influenced by many factors including the family and social environment, developmental competencies, and secondary stressors (Margolin et al. 2010). Children and adolescents who are physically abused or exposed to parents' domestic violence often experience pervasive traumatic stress and can develop PTSD (Becker et al. 2010; Margolin and Vickerman 2007). Childhood sexual abuse can result in PTSD, other psychiatric conditions, and have long-term adverse health consequences including alcohol and drug abuse, increased risk for HIV/AIDS, and chronic pain (Jonas et al. 2011; Lalor and McElvaney 2010; Mimiaga et al. 2009; Arnow 2004). The often repeating or ongoing nature of exposure to family violence can lead to difficulties in several areas of functioning (for example, decreased cognitive performance, risk-taking behaviors, and delinquency) and result in PTSD as well as other anxiety and mood disorders (Margolin et al. 2010). Traumatic events that can lead to PTSD include not only extraordinary events such as natural or man-made disasters, but also events that occur within families that are capable of causing death, injury, or threaten the physical integrity of a child or members of their family (Margolin and Vickerman 2007). Examples include child sexual abuse, physical abuse, neglect, or witnessing domestic abuse of a parent. About 30–50% of sexually abused children meet criteria for a PTSD diagnosis (Maikovich et al. 2009). Studies have shown that domestic violence occurs in the homes of about 30% of youth living with two parents (McDonald et al. 2006). About 5–10% of children in the United States are victims of severe physical abuse each year (Margolin and Vickerman 2007). Children and adolescents can be exposed to multiple forms of family violence as well as community violence (Margolin and Gordis 2000; Crusto et al. 2010).

It is not completely understood why some persons exposed to trauma early in life are profoundly affected while others are not. Genetic factors associated with PTSD are discussed later in this chapter. Studies of how children and adolescents cope with traumatic events have identified not only vulnerability factors (for example, trauma at a younger developmental age or having a positive family history of PTSD), but also protective factors such as having a healthy family environment and better parenting (Graham-Bermann et al. 2009). Based upon studies conducted in diverse cultures, there is growing appreciation for the remarkable resilience often demonstrated by children and adolescents who are exposed to trauma (Caffo and Belaise 2003). For example, higher family education levels and improved family functioning (measured using the McMaster Family Assessment Device) were found to protect against

PTSD among Jewish Israeli and Palestinian adolescents exposed to political violence (Al-Krenawi et al. 2009). In a study of former Ugandan child soldiers, Klasen et al. (2010) found that post-traumatic resilience was associated with lower exposure to domestic violence, better socioeconomic situation in the family, more perceived spiritual support, and lower guilt cognitions. Other important aspects of interpersonal violence and PTSD (for example, physical or sexual assault among women) are further discussed in Chapter 2.

COGNITION AND MEMORY IN THE DEVELOPMENT OR MAINTENANCE OF PTSD

In the decades that have passed since PTSD was first included as a diagnostic entity in DSM-III, a large literature has emerged on psychological and cognitive factors that may have a role in the development or maintenance of PTSD. Several psychological models of PTSD have been proposed including conditioning theory, cognitive theory, emotional processing theory, and schema theory, to name a few. Psychological models of PTSD are refined over time through clinical experience, through discussion and debate among experts in the field, and by testing psychological theory against observations from psychological and neurobiological research including genetic and brain imaging studies. In this section, an overview of research findings and theoretical models is shared from the clinical psychology and neuropsychology literature that have strived to ground conceptual understandings of PTSD in cognition, memory, and related factors.

In developing theoretical models for PTSD, some authors have focused on fear conditioning (Keane et al. 1985; Kilpatrick et al. 1985; Kolb 1989). Conditioning theories are consistent with classic psychological models of learning and conditioning (Friedman 1997). According to such theories, persons exposed to a life-threatening experience may become conditioned to stimuli that were present during the trauma. These stimuli, including previously neutral stimuli, subsequently elicit high levels of anxiety (Cahill and Foa 2007). As a result of higher order conditioning and generalization of stimuli, a variety of situations may then induce fear.

Neurobiological research and concepts of activated fear networks provide some support for conditioning theories of PTSD. Animal studies and brain imaging studies in human volunteers have identified neurological circuitry that plays a role in the processing of stressful or fearful stimuli (Friedman and Karam 2009). The neuroimaging and neuroanatomy of PTSD have been reviewed by Rauch and Drevets (2009) and Robinson and Shergill (2011). The amygdala, which is activated by stressful or fear-raising stimuli, has outputs to the hippocampus, which helps mediate the consolidation of memory. The locus coeruleus and hypothalamus also have a role in the processing of fear reactions. In persons with PTSD, the normal disinhibition of the amygdala by the medial prefrontal cortex is disrupted and, as a result, ambiguous stimuli are more likely to be misinterpreted as threatening (Charney 2004; Friedman and Karam 2009). Neuroimaging studies have demonstrated that, when PTSD patients are presented with auditory or visual stimuli that remind them of their traumatic experience, they exhibit increased amygdala activation and reduced activation of the prefrontal cortex (Kaufman et al. 2004). These findings have prompted extended discussion about whether PTSD should be classified as a stress-related fear circuitry disorder (Friedman and Karam 2009).

Studies of cognitive aspects of PTSD have informed psychological models for the disorder. Cognitions refer to information structures that result from perception, learning, reasoning, or memory and include representations of stimuli and responses (Huppert et al. 2009). Cognitions can be contrasted with physiological anxiety symptoms. Cognitive processes are mechanisms that underlie cognitions involved in the detection, encoding, storage, retrieval, and utilization of information (Huppert et al. 2009). They range from automatic processes used without effort or awareness to strategic processes that are used purposefully with awareness.

A variety of memory disturbances have been observed in persons with PTSD including changes in memory capacity, the content of trauma-related memories, and certain memory processes (Brewin 2011; Rubin et al. 2008). Although results from experimental studies and clinical research indicate that some memory changes are likely to be "epiphenomena" in that they reflect the effects of PTSD, experimental evidence also supports a causal role for some memory disturbances (Brewin 2011). In a recent comprehensive review of memory disturbances in PTSD, Brewin (2011) concluded that verbal memory deficits, negative conceptual knowledge of self, avoidance or suppression of memories, and negative interpretation of memory symptoms are likely to have a role in the development or maintenance of PTSD. These memory disturbances are not necessarily specific to PTSD. However, there are other memory disturbances specific to PTSD that likely have a causal role (Brewin 2011). These include difficulties with integration of the trauma with self-identify, impairment in voluntary retrieval of traumatic memories (i.e., difficulty with deliberate retrieval of contextualized memories of the traumatic event), and increased frequency of sensation-related memories or flashbacks (Brewin 2011). Persons with PTSD suffer from disorganized, fragmented memories of the trauma and from vivid intrusive images triggered by a wide variety of stimuli (Rubin et al. 2008; Brewin 2011).

Cognitive theories of PTSD assume that cognitions play a causal role in the development or maintenance of the disorder through cognitive biases in which patients are more apt to focus on negative information or ignore positive information and to negatively interpret ambiguous information as a threat, that is, negative evaluations of stimuli (Huppert et al. 2009). Such theories also assume that people differ in the extent to which they focus on negative or positive information and that a tendency to focus on negative information increases vulnerability to anxiety. As an example, in tests of explicit memory, persons with and without PTSD are asked to remember word lists, and then the numbers of threat versus nonthreat words recalled are examined. In tests of implicit memory, a memory bias for threat information may be inferred from greater recall or use of threat-related words as compared with nonthreat-related words (Huppert et al. 2009). Although persons with PTSD have been found to have changes in explicit memory, an implicit memory bias has not been consistently identified in PTSD patients (Brewin 2011). Experimental studies have indicated that persons with PTSD are more likely to complete sentences with words that have threat meanings, which is consistent with a negative interpretation bias (Kimble et al. 2002). Studies have also shown an attentional bias for trauma-related cues in PTSD patients (Foa et al. 1991; McNally 1998). Persons who suffer from PTSD are also more apt to view the world as being more dangerous or threatening, than persons without the disorder, and they may also hold negative views about their competence or ability to cope (Ehlers et al. 2005). In their cognitive model of PTSD, which has several features in common with emotional processing theory (Foa and Kozak 1985), Ehlers and Clark (2000) posited that persons with chronic PTSD process a traumatic event (or its consequences) in a way that gives rise to a sense of current threat.

In addition to conditioning theories and cognitive theory, emotional processing theory has also been widely used to account for why some people exposed to trauma develop PTSD and why some trauma survivors do not recover from their symptoms (Foa and Kozak 1985; Cahill and Foa 2007). One premise of emotional processing theory is that PTSD and other anxiety disorders reflect the presence of pathological fear structures embedded in memory (Cahill and Foa 2007). According to this theory, fear structures include interrelated representations of feared stimuli, fear responses, and meanings that are associated with them. These fear structures are activated by information in the environment that matches information in the fear structure, which produces the cognitive, behavioral, and physiological reactions seen in PTSD (Foa and Kozak 1985; Cahill and Foa 2007). Emotional processing theory posits that chronic PTSD represents an inability to adequately process the traumatic memory. The theory emphasizes that persons with PTSD avoid trauma-related thoughts and reminders as a way of coping with the distress associated with reexperiencing the trauma, and that avoidance may also impede natural recovery from the disorder in some persons. Although emotional processing theory has several parallels with conditioning theories of PTSD, emotional processing theory incorporates associations between feared stimuli and responses and the meanings associated with both stimuli and responses (Cahill and Foa 2007).

Other authors have extended personality theory and theories from social psychology to try to account for the psychological effects of traumatic exposures (Horowitz 1986; Epstein 1991). These theories—referred to as schema theories—utilize the concept of schemas, or core assumptions and beliefs that guide the perception and interpretation of information. Schema theories offer several important insights including the observation that traumatic experiences may alter a person's core beliefs about the nature of the world (for example, trauma victims may no longer view the world as benign or that people can be trusted). However, other theories (for example, emotional processing theory and cognitive theory) are better able to account for why cognitive-behavioral therapies for PTSD are effective in alleviating symptoms of the disorder (Cahill and Foa 2007).

BIOLOGICAL MODELS OF PTSD

Previous authors have noted that the biological correlates of PTSD are similar to those of chronic stress (Friedman and McEwen 2004; Schnurr and Green 2004). The effects of traumatic exposures or chronic stress on the hypothalamic-pituitary-adrenal (HPA) axis and the autonomic nervous system have been examined in clinical studies and in animal models. Acute stress prompts a cascade of neurohormonal events in humans and animals including release of hypothalamic corticotrophin-releasing hormone (CRH) into the pituitary portal system and increased turnover of norepinephrine in terminal projection regions of the locus coeruleus (Jacobsen et al. 2001). Studies of healthy adults have associated stress and anxiety with increased cortisol, plasma and urinary norepinephrine, epinephrine, and their metabolites (Bedi and Arora 2007; Lader 1974). Adrenal corticosteroids, sometimes referred to as glucocorticoids, are released by the adrenal cortex in response to adrenocorticotropic hormone (ACTH) produced in the anterior pituitary gland. One of the major glucocorticoids is cortisol. The production and secretion of ACTH by the pituitary is stimulated by hypothalamic CRH. A feedback loop exists such that glucocorticoids secreted by the adrenal gland inhibit CRH secretion by the hypothalamus. The hypothalamus, amygdala, hippocampus, and other brain tissues contain cortisol receptors (de Kloet and Reul 1987). Sympathetic activation and other physiological reactions to acute stress are contained or shut down through negative feedback inhibition by cortisol. As noted by Yehuda (2000), the biology of the acute stress response is not necessarily the same as the biology of PTSD.

Persons with PTSD have been reported to have dysregulation of the HPA axis with higher or lower cortisol levels and increased numbers of glucocorticoid receptors (Schnurr and Green 2004). Individual differences in number or functional activity of glucocorticoid receptors could account for why everyone does not respond to extreme stress in the same manner (Yehuda 2000). Clinical studies have found that cerebrospinal fluid levels of CRH are elevated in patients with PTSD, which is consistent with increased activity of the HPA system in the central nervous system (Rohleder and Karl 2006; Baker et al. 2005; Bremner et al. 1997). In studies of urinary cortisol excretion in patients with PTSD, urinary cortisol concentrations have been reported to be elevated in some, but not all studies (Rohleder and Karl 2006; Yehuda et al. 1993). Research findings of the effects of chronic stress or of PTSD on HPA axis function have varied by study population and experimental design (Jacobsen et al. 2001). Both elevated and reduced cortisol secretion have been reported in persons with PTSD (Maes et al. 1998; Mason et al. 1988). A recent meta-analysis by Meewisse et al. (2007), which summarized findings from 37 studies, found that persons with PTSD had significantly lower levels of plasma or serum cortisol than persons not exposed to trauma, although overall results were highly heterogeneous. Although findings to date have been inconsistent, altered cortisol levels among persons with PTSD could contribute to a higher or lower risk of other health conditions including diseases affected by immune function and those mediated by chronic inflammation (Schnurr and Green 2004). In addition, increased levels of CRH in the brain, particularly in the amygdala, may mediate risk for substance abuse and dependence in people who suffer from PTSD (Jacobsen et al. 2001).

Persons with PTSD also exhibit elevated basal adrenergic levels and heightened adrenergic reactivity (Schnurr and Green 2004). Norepinephrine turnover increases in the locus coeruleus, hypothalamus, amygdala, and cerebral cortex during chronic stress (Jacobsen et al. 2001). Cardiovascular alterations associated with autonomic arousal and cardiovascular health outcomes have been reported to be associated with PTSD or wartime traumatic exposures (McFarlane 2010; Boscarino 2004). Persons suffering from PTSD and chronic PTSD exhibit increases in basal heart rate and blood pressure as well as increased heart rate and blood pressure in response to stimuli such as loud sounds and visual slides that remind them of the trauma (Gerardi et al. 1994; Keane et al. 1998; Bedi and Arora 2007; Kleim et al. 2010; Gutner et al. 2010). These research findings are consistent with increased sympathetic activity among persons with PTSD (Bedi and Arora 2007; Cohen et al. 2000). In clinical studies involving small sample groups of veterans, plasma norepinephrine and 24-hour urine norepinephrine levels have been reported to be elevated among veterans with PTSD as compared to those without PTSD (Mason et al. 1988). Elevated catecholamine levels cause downregulation of β- and α_2-adrenergic receptors (Friedman 1997). Dysregulation of the HPA axis and chronic overstimulation of the autonomic nervous system may contribute to the increases in blood pressure and lipid levels that have been observed in PTSD patients. In addition to the HPA axis and the catecholamine system, at least three other systems are involved in PTSD. These include the endogenous opioid systems, the thyroid, and the immune system (Friedman 1997). Biological models of PTSD should ideally take into account interactions between biological systems and dynamic changes over time since biological alterations in PTSD may evolve over time (Yehuda 2000).

Immunologic Changes in PTSD

The immune system, which participates in the overall preservation of homeostasis, interacts with the HPA axis in a bidirectional fashion (Chrousos 1995). Immune cells secrete cytokines (small protein or peptide cell-signaling molecules) that act on other immune cells and tissues throughout the body including those in the central nervous system (Dougall and Baum 2004). The release of cytokines can result in many signs and symptoms including fatigue, fever, depressed mood, and inflammation. Cortisol modifies the vast cytokine system through its interaction with cellular glucocorticoid receptors (Vidovic et al. 2007).

Observations that persons with PTSD have altered cortisol levels have prompted studies of immune function and mediators of inflammation in persons exposed to trauma and extreme stress. Most studies of immune function in persons suffering from PTSD have examined numbers and percentages of circulating immune cells (Rohleder and Karl 2006). Conflicting findings have been reported from studies of B and T lymphocyte counts among persons with PTSD, which may be partly due to the nature of the traumatic exposures (Boscarino 2004; Woods et al. 2005; Kawamura et al. 2001; Wilson et al. 1999; Vidovic et al. 2007). In a study of Croatian War veterans, Vidovic et al. (2007) observed higher lymphocyte counts in PTSD patients than in healthy controls ($p = 0.007$). Lymphocyte glucocorticoid receptor expression was also positively related to the number of years since the traumatic exposure (Vidovic et al. 2007). In addition to studies of lymphocyte counts among persons who developed PTSD following severe stressors such as combat exposures, there is a sizeable literature on alterations of immunity following less severe stressors, as reviewed by Dougall and Baum (2004) and others.

Some studies of PTSD and immune function have employed functional assays of humoral or cellular immunity such as skin tests of delayed-type hypersensitivity reactions and in vitro tests of natural killer (NK) cell activity (Rohleder and Karl 2006). Researchers have found that NK cells obtained from PTSD patients are less efficient at lysing specific target cells (Ironson et al. 1997; Kawamura et al. 2001; Mosnaim et al. 1993; Inoue-Sakurai et al. 2000; Gotovac et al. 2010), although conflicting results have also been reported (Delahanty et al. 1997; Laudenslager et al. 1998). In a study by Mosnaim et al. (1993), decreased NK cell activity was only observed in cells obtained from PTSD patients after an in vitro challenge with methinonine-enkephalin.

Results obtained from other studies, in which antigens were applied to the skin of PTSD patients and the local immune response measured, have suggested that persons with PTSD may have increased cell-mediated immunity (Watson et al. 1993; Altemus et al. 2003).

Studies that have assessed immune function overactivity in persons exposed to trauma may be particularly informative for understanding biological pathways that lead to important health outcomes such as chronic pain, autoimmune conditions, and certain chronic diseases. These include studies that have examined concentrations of circulating mediators of inflammation such as interleukin-1 (IL-1), interleukin-6 (IL-6), C-reactive protein, and other inflammatory mediators (Miller et al. 2001; Tucker et al. 2004; Spivak et al. 1997; Maes et al. 1999; Baker et al. 2001; Gill et al. 2008). Tucker et al. (2004) observed higher serum concentrations of IL-1β and lower soluble interleukin-2 receptors (IL-2R) in 58 PTSD patients compared with 21 controls. In a pilot study of 15 PTSD patients and 8 controls with musculoskeletal injuries who were at least three months postinjury, Miller et al. (2001) found a positive relationship between serum IL-6 receptor levels and PTSD severity. Levels of C-reactive protein were also positively related to measures of psychological distress in the PTSD patients (Miller et al. 2001). Spivak et al. (1997) assessed serum levels of IL-1β and soluble IL-2R in 19 male patients with combat-related PTSD and 19 age- and sex-matched healthy controls. Levels of serum IL-1β, but not soluble IL-2R, were significantly higher in the PTSD patients than in the controls ($p < 0.001$). A correlation was observed between IL-1β levels and duration of PTSD symptoms but not with severity of PTSD (Spivak et al. 1997). Maes et al. (1999) examined the inflammatory response system in patients with PTSD using measurements of serum IL-6, soluble IL-6R, sgp130 (the IL-6 signal-transducing protein), an endogenous IL-1R antagonist, CC16 (an endogenous anticytokine), and CD8 (T-lymphocyte suppressor cell antigen). Serum concentrations of IL-6 and soluble IL-6R, but not sgp130, soluble IL-RA, CC16, or CD8, were significantly higher in PTSD patients than in healthy controls. No significant relationships were observed between serum IL-6 or soluble IL-6R and severity of PTSD. Gill et al. (2008) observed higher levels of IL-6 and tumor necrosis factor-α in a sample of women with PTSD than in female controls. Baker et al. (2001) examined plasma and cerebrospinal fluid IL-6 levels in a study of 11 veterans with PTSD and 8 age- and sex-matched healthy controls. Mean cerebrospinal fluid IL-6 levels were higher in

PTSD patients than in controls ($p = 0.05$) but no differences were observed in plasma IL-6 levels between patients and controls (Baker et al. 2001). Taken overall, findings from these studies suggest that PTSD is associated with increased secretion of proinflammatory cytokines, including IL-6, which may be due to disinhibition of the inflammatory response. Although findings across studies have not always been consistent, these differences may be partly due to the nature of the psychological trauma and the duration of time elapsed since the traumatic event (Dougall and Baum 2004). Inflammatory mediators such as C-reactive protein are further discussed in Chapters 7 and 8.

Studies of immune function in persons with PTSD may help to clarify biological pathways that account for gender disparities in trauma-related adverse health conditions, including conditions that are more prevalent in women than in men, or which only occur among women (Gill et al. 2005). Several autoimmune conditions have been found to be more prevalent among women and there is continuing interest in clarifying whether persons with PTSD have a higher risk of autoimmune conditions (Kimerling 2004). Neylan et al. (2011) examined circulating monocytes obtained from male and female PTSD patients and age- and sex-matched controls using gene expression microarray analysis. The researchers observed differential patterns of gene expression on monocytes obtained from male and female subjects (Neylan et al. 2011; O'Donovan et al. 2011).

Although dysregulation of the HPA axis, changes in cortisol levels, and downregulation of genes associated with glucocorticoid receptors may account for immunologic changes in PTSD (O'Donovan et al. 2011), other mechanisms may also have a role. For example, increased alcohol consumption and cigarette smoking, associated with PTSD in clinical and epidemiologic studies, have adverse effects on the immune system (Dougall and Baum 2004). Genetic or epigenetic mechanisms may also play a role (Schmidt et al. 2011). Preliminary evidence from a study by Uddin et al. (2010) suggested that PTSD may lead to alterations in immune function by reducing methylation levels of immune-related genes. The association of PTSD risk with maternal PTSD is also consistent with epigenetic explanations (Yehuda and Bierer 2009). Additional studies are needed to confirm epigenetic hypotheses about the pathogenesis of PTSD, however.

Genetics of PTSD

The hypothesis of a heritable contribution to PTSD susceptibility was first examined in a series of studies of family members of individuals with PTSD or who had been exposed to traumatic events. These studies primarily took two forms: (1) family studies in which either the parent or child had been exposed to trauma, and (2) twin studies in which the twins were discordant for traumatic exposures.

The initial family studies by Davidson et al. (1985, 1989) examined the presence of developmental and psychological disorders in the children of Vietnam veterans with PTSD, and suggested that familial tendencies toward PTSD and other anxiety disorders may exist. Subsequent studies identified transgenerational trends in PTSD occurrence among Cambodian refugees (Sack et al. 1995), Holocaust survivors (Yehuda et al. 1998, 2001, 2002), and survivors of the World Trade Center terrorist attacks (Yehuda et al. 2005). In these studies, adult children of parents with PTSD were more likely to develop PTSD than children of parents without PTSD. A physiological associate of susceptibility (salivary cortisol) was also examined in two of the studies (Yehuda et al. 2002, 2005).

There have been many studies of PTSD in twins. One of the first (Skre et al. 1993) was performed in a small set of 40 co-twins of anxiety disorder probands and 32 nonproband co-twins who did not suffer from psychosis. Findings of a higher prevalence of PTSD among monozygotic than dizygotic co-twins suggested a heritable contribution to PTSD. This finding was followed by a series of studies developed within the Vietnam Era Twin (VET) Registry (Eisen et al. 1987). The VET Registry was created during 1983–1986 and ultimately enrolled a total of 7,375 twin pairs (male/male) who had been born between 1939 and 1955 that had served in the military during the Vietnam War era. Additional data were gathered from this cohort during the 1993 Harvard Twin Study of Drug Abuse and Dependence. Early work in the VET Registry estimated that 13–34% of the variance in risk of symptoms is due to genetic factors (True et al. 1993). A second study found that a total of 34.9% of genetic variability in PTSD was due to additive genetic contributions that were either PTSD-specific (13.6%) or shared with generalized anxiety disorder and/or panic disorder (21.3%) (Chantarujikapong et al. 2001). This finding was supported by an estimate that approximately 58% of the genetic variance in PTSD is accounted for by additive genetic contributions shared by major depression. This shared contribution was demonstrated by an increased correlation coefficient for the association between major depression and PTSD among monozygotic twins, relative to that observed among dizygotic twins

(Koenen et al. 2003, 2008). Similarly, evaluations of the genetic contributions to PTSD within the context of substance abuse disorders estimated that 20% of the genetic variation in PTSD was PTSD-specific, 15.3% was shared in common with alcohol and drug abuse (Xian et al. 2000), and shared contributions accounted for 63% of the association between PTSD and nicotine dependence (Koenen et al. 2005). Evaluations of heritability within the context of traditional psychological risk factors found that familial effects were somewhat mediated by the characteristics of the trauma received, and by preexisting proband pathologies (Koenen et al. 2002). Among PTSD probands and their combat-unexposed co-twins, higher prevalence of neurological characteristics (neurological soft signs, reduced hippocampal volume, and abnormal cavum septum pellucidum), relative to non-PTSD twin pairs, provided additional evidence of familial susceptibility to PTSD (Pitman et al. 2006; Gurvits et al. 2006; Gilbertson et al. 2002; May et al. 2004).

Smaller studies have been performed outside of the VET Registry. In a predominantly female sample of twin pairs from the urban Vancouver region, the PTSD heritability among twins concordant for trauma exposure was estimated to be 0.28 to 0.38 (Stein et al. 2002). Additional evidence of heritability was provided by a study of a small sample of 19 twin pairs that found inferior neurocognitive performance within the PTSD twin pairs. This suggested that familial contributions to cognition could act as a protective mechanism among those with above-average cognitive performance (Gilbertson et al. 2006). In contrast, a later imaging study failed to detect evidence of a heritable gray matter reduction that would indicate a familial vulnerability to PTSD (Kasai et al. 2008). Psychometric evaluation (including the Mississippi PTSD Scale) also did not reveal evidence of a predisposing psychological factor among the co-twins of combat-exposed veterans with PTSD (Gilbertson et al. 2010).

Genetic Association Studies

Substantial work has been done to evaluate associations between PTSD and polymorphisms in genes associated with dopamine and serotonin metabolism. Somewhat less research has been performed exploring associations with variations in brain-derived neurotrophic factor (BDNF), glucocorticoid receptor, apolipoprotein-E (APOE), neuropeptide Y (NPY), FK506 binding protein 5 (FKPB5), cannabinoid receptor 1 (CNR1), gamma-aminobutyric acid receptor subunit alpha-2 (GABRA2), catechol-O-methyl transferase (COMT), regulator of G-protein signaling 2 (RGS2), dysbindin, cholinergic receptor nicotinic alpha-5 gene (CHRNA5), and pituitary adenylate cyclase 1 (PAC1) genes. The dopamine D2 receptor gene (DRD2) features a *Taq* I polymorphism. In a series of studies of persons suffering from alcohol or drug abuse, the D2A1 allele of DRD2 was found to have a highly increased prevalence among individuals with PTSD and other disorders (Comings et al. 1991, 1996; Young et al. 2002; Lawford et al. 2006). These results were not replicated in studies by Gelernter et al. (1999), Voisey (2009), and Bailey (2010). However, Voisey (2009) did identify an association between PTSD status and the 957C>T synonymous polymorphism (rs6277) of DRD2. The 957C>T variant was later shown to be associated with fear conditioning and the aversive priming effect (Huertas et al. 2010).

A polymorphism in the dopamine D4 receptor gene (DRD4) has also been demonstrated to be associated with PTSD symptoms. In a study of flood survivors (Dragan and Oniszczenko 2009), the exon III polymorphism was associated with avoidance/numbing category symptoms and with total symptom intensity.

The dopamine transporter contains an untranslated polymorphic variable number tandem repeat (VNTR) region in the SCL6A3 3' region. It is hypothesized that effects of this VNTR are exhibited during mRNA transcription, or through correlation (linkage disequilibrium) with a separate site. Segman et al. (2002) identified an association between the 9-repeat allele of this VNTR and PTSD, such that PTSD sufferers carried it at a significantly higher prevalence. This finding was replicated in a study of children affected by Hurricane Katrina (Drury et al. 2009) and Brazilian urban violence victims (Valente et al. 2011), but not in a study of earthquake victims (Bailey et al. 2010).

Finally, a study of the –1021C/T polymorphism of the dopamine beta-hydroxylase (DBH) gene and plasma DBH activity found that the CC genotype conferred the greatest DBH activity, TT the least activity, and CT an intermediate level (Mustapic et al. 2007). Within each genotype, veterans with PTSD had lower activity than non-PTSD veterans. However, this comparison was statistically significant only within the CC genotype. A second study (Tang et al. 2010) replicated the observed association between genotype and serum DBH activity.

The serotonin transporter gene (SERT, 5-HTTLPR) contains a polymorphism in its promoter region. This most commonly occurs in short and long forms (14 and 16 repeats, respectively), but several additional alleles have been recognized (Nakamura et al. 2000). The polymorphism is associated with anxiety disorders (Lesch et al. 1996) and increased amygdalar response to fearful stimuli (Hariri et al. 2002); the *s/s* genotype was found to be more common among PTSD sufferers (Lee et al. 2005), with evidence of gene-environment interactions (Kilpatrick et al. 2007; Koenen et al. 2009; Xie et al. 2009; Kolassa et al. 2010). Other studies with contradictory findings found the *l/l* allele to be more common among motor vehicle accident victims with PTSD (Thakur et al. 2009) and among PTSD sufferers in the general population (Grabe et al. 2009). Another study failed to detect any association (Valente et al. 2011; Mellman et al. 2009; Sayin et al. 2010).

A small number of studies have also evaluated the association between PTSD and the serotonin 2A receptor gene (5-HTR2A) –1438A/G polymorphism. These have provided generally concordant results, suggesting that the G allele (Mellman et al. 2009) or GG genotype (Lee et al. 2007) occurred more frequently in PTSD patients than controls.

Four single nucleotide polymorphisms (SNPs) in the FKBP5 gene locus were found to interact with cumulative childhood trauma (Binder et al. 2008) and were associated with peritraumatic dissociation among children with acute medical injuries (Koenen et al. 2005). The findings of a gene-environment interaction were later replicated among African-Americans, but not among persons of European descent (Xie et al. 2010; Boscarino et al. 2011). These results are intriguing, given FKBP5's role as a glucocorticoid receptor regulator of stress proteins such as hsp90, and participant in the glucocorticoid receptor complex (Binder 2009).

The gene for COMT, which supports the inactivation of catecholamines such as dopamine, has a functional substitution Val158Met. This polymorphism results in lower enzyme activity, and a gene-environment interaction has been observed such that Met/Met genotypes have a high risk of PTSD regardless of their exposure to trauma (Kolassa et al. 2010). This was supported by evidence that the rs4680 SNP of COMT is associated with PTSD (Boscarino et al. 2011; Valente et al. 2011).

The RGS2 gene polymorphism rs4606 has been shown to be associated with generalized anxiety disorder (Koenen et al. 2009) and with PTSD symptoms in the presence of high stress exposure and low social support (Amstadter et al. 2009a). In the same sample of Florida residents of areas affected by the 2004 hurricanes, RGS2 variation was also associated with suicidal ideation (Amstadter et al. 2009b).

Several additional genes have been evaluated for association with PTSD in a small number of studies. In a study of childhood trauma exposures, the GABRA2 gene was also found to be subject to an interaction with cumulative trauma (Nelson et al. 2009). One haplotype of the CNR1 gene was associated with PTSD (Lu et al. 2008), as were variants in the CHRNA5 gene (Boscarino et al. 2011) and dysbindin gene (DTNBP1; Voisey et al. 2010). In a small study of 54 veterans with PTSD, the APOE2 allele was associated with worse symptoms of reexperiencing and with worse memory function; however, no differences were noted in association with the APOE4 allele (Freeman et al. 2005). Finally, the PAC1 SNP rs2267735, located within a predicted estrogen response element, was observed to be associated with PTSD symptoms among females (Ressler et al. 2011).

The N363S and *BclI* polymorphisms of the glucocorticoid receptor gene were initially found to have no association with PTSD (Bachmann et al. 2005). However, evidence of an association has since been reported, such that individuals homozygous for the *BclI* allele have increased PTSD symptoms (Hauer et al. 2011).

No association was identified between PTSD and the Leu7Pro polymorphism of the NPY gene (Lappalainen et al. 2002), or the Val66Met, G-712A, and C270T polymorphisms of the BDNF gene (Valente et al. 2011; Lee et al. 2006; Zhang et al. 2006).

In considering the heritability of PTSD, it is important to consider the heritability of exposure to the prerequisite traumatizing factor. For this reason, we provide a brief summary of this parallel path of research. In a twin study based in the VET Registry, the heritability of volunteering for service was estimated to be 0.36. A total of 57% of the additive genetic contributions to volunteering for service and experiencing combat exposure were shared between the two factors (Lyons et al. 1993). In a general population twin study, approximately 5–11% of the correlation between personality characteristics and trauma exposure was accounted for by genetic factors (Jang et al. 2003). A more recent meta-analysis found that the C-521T polymorphism of DRD4 is associated with the personality characteristics of novelty seeking and impulsivity (Munafo et al. 2008). These results support the need for additional research to fully untangle the role of heritability in the development of PTSD.

Gene Expression

Few studies to date have studied gene expression in PTSD. Segman et al. (2005) performed a prospective study of trauma survivors who had been admitted to an emergency room following a traumatic event. Hierarchical cluster analysis of gene expression at four months perfectly separated participants who did not meet DSM-IV criteria for acute and chronic PTSD at either one month or four months after the event from those who met criteria at both time points. A total of 656 of 4,512 transcripts were significantly differentially expressed between these two groups during the four month follow-up period; when time points were considered separately, 574 transcripts from the initial (emergency room) blood draw and 408 at month four were differentially expressed. More genes than expected demonstrated a correlation between four month expression and total Impact of Event Scale (IES) score, as well as the three IES symptom cluster subscores. Similar results were observed for gene expression at the ER time point. The set of differentially expressed genes had a strong representation of genes expressed in amygdalar, hippocampal, and HPA axis regions.

A subsequent study (Zieker et al. 2007) examined the expression of 277 PBMC transcripts focused on stress and immune responses. After comparing transcript expression between the patients and controls, five upregulated and 14 downregulated genes were identified that were, as a group, related to reactive oxygen species (ROS) metabolism. This suggested that disturbances in the oxidative stress system and associated immune factors may contribute to PTSD symptoms. In a study of individuals exposed to the World Trade Center attacks, differential expression of genes pertinent to the HPA axis, brain and immune cells, and signal transduction was observed (Yehuda et al. 2009). Additional support was provided by recent findings of increased activity in immune-related pathways in females, but not males (Neylan et al. 2011). These studies of gene expression in PTSD have been based on small samples, raising questions of statistical power and generalizability. However, their results are relatively consistent in suggesting perturbations in the expression of genes relating to the stress and immune response systems. Further studies building on these findings will add greatly to our understanding of the natural history of PTSD at the molecular, individual, and environmental levels.

SUMMARY AND CONCLUSIONS

This chapter has summarized several key areas of PTSD research including: (1) studies of risk factors for PTSD in children, adolescents, and adults; (2) psychological and biological models of PTSD; (3) immunologic changes associated with the disorder; and (4) genetic findings from studies of PTSD patients. Findings from psychological and biological studies as well as refinements in diagnostic criteria contribute to translational clinical research that has identified effective psychological and medical treatments for PTSD. This includes group or individual psychotherapy (for example, cognitive-behavioral therapy) and pharmacotherapy, such as the use of selective serotonin reuptake inhibitors (Karlin et al. 2010). Cognitive-behavioral therapy helps patients to address their traumatic memories and distorted cognitions by providing education about the nature of PTSD and stress responses and helping the individual with the integration of the traumatic events. Education about skills for anxiety self-management is also vital. Studies have also shown that family support and support from peers play an important part in recovery.

REFERENCES

Al-Krenawi A, Graham JR, Kanat-Maymon Y. 2009. Analysis of trauma exposure, symptomatology and functioning in Jewish Israeli and Palestinian adolescents. *Br J Psychiatry.* 195:427–432.

Altemus M, Cloitre M, Dhabhar FS. 2003. Enhanced cellular immune response in women with PTSD related to childhood abuse. *Am J Psychiatry.* 160:1705–1707.

Amstadter AB, Koenen KC, Ruggiero KJ, et al. 2009a. Variant in RGS2 moderates posttraumatic stress symptoms following potentially traumatic event exposure. *Journal of Anxiety Disorders.* 23:369–373.

Amstadter AB, Koenen KC, Ruggiero KJ, et al. 2009b. Variation in RGS2 is associated with suicidal ideation in an epidemiological study of adults exposed to the 2004 Florida hurricanes. *Arch Suicide Res.* 13:349–357.

Arnow BA. 2004. Relationships between childhood maltreatment, adult health and psychiatric outcomes, and medical utilization. *J Clin Psychiatry.* 65(Suppl 12):10–15.

Bachmann AW, Sedgley TL, Jackson RV, et al. 2005. Glucocorticoid receptor polymorphisms and post-traumatic stress disorder. *Psychoneuroendocrinology.* 30:297–306.

Bailey JN, Goenjian AK, Noble EP, Walling DP. 2010. PTSD and dopaminergic genes, DRD2 and DAT, in multigenerational families exposed to the Spitak earthquake. *Psychiatry Research.* 178:507–510.

Baker DG, Ekhator NN, Kasckow JW, et al. 2001. Plasma and cerebrospinal fluid interleukin-6 concentrations in posttraumatic stress disorder. *Neuroimmunomodulation.* 9:209–217.

Baker DG, Ekhator NN, Kasckow JW, et al. 2005. Higher levels of basal serial CSF cortisol in combat veterans with posttraumatic stress disorder. *Am J Psychiatry.* 162:992–994.

Becker KD, Stuewig J, McCloskey LA. 2010. Traumatic stress symptoms of women exposed to different forms of childhood victimization and intimate partner violence. *J Interpers Violence.* 25:1699–715.

Bedi US, Arora R. 2007. Cardiovascular manifestations of posttraumatic stress disorder. *J National Med Assoc.* 99:642–649.

Binder EB. 2009. The role of FKBP5, a co-chaperone of the glucocorticoid receptor in the pathogenesis and therapy of affective and anxiety disorders. *Psychoneuroendocrinology.* 345:S186–S195.

Binder E, Bradley R, Liu W, et al. 2008. Association of FKBP5 polymorphisms and childhood abuse with risk of posttraumatic stress disorder symptoms in adults. *JAMA.* 299:1291–1305.

Boscarino JA. 2004. Posttraumatic stress disorder and physical illness. Results from clinical and epidemiologic studies. *Ann NY Acad Sci.* 1032:141–153.

Boscarino JA, Erlich PM, Hoffman SN, et al. 2011. Association of FKBP5, COMT and CHRNA5 polymorphisms with PTSD among outpatients at risk for PTSD. *Psychiatry Research.* 188:173–174.

Bremner JD, Licinio J, Darnell A, et al. 1997. Elevated CSF corticotropin-releasing factor concentrations in posttraumatic stress disorder. *Am J Psychiatry.* 154:624–629.

Breslan N, Davis GC. 1992. Posttraumatic stress disorder in an urban population of young adults: risk factors for chronicity. *Am J Psychiatry.* 49:671–679.

Brewin CR. 2011. The nature and significance of memory disturbance in posttraumatic stress disorder. *Annu Rev Clin Psychol.* 7:203–227.

Caffo E, Belaise C. 2003. Psychological aspects of traumatic injury in children and adolescents. *Child Adolesc Psychiatr Clin N Am.* 12:493–535.

Cahill SP, Foa EB. 2007. Psychological theories of PTSD. In: Friedman MJ, Keane TM, Resick PA, editors. *Handbook of PTSD: Science and practice.* New York: The Gulford Press: 55–77.

Charney DS. 2004. Psychobiological mechanisms of resilience and vulnerability: implications for the successful adaptation to extreme stress. *Am J Psychiatry.* 161:195–216.

Chantarujikapong SI, Scherrer JF, Xian H, et al. 2001. A twin study of generalized anxiety disorder symptoms, panic disorder symptoms and post-traumatic stress disorder in men. *Psychiatry Research.* 103:133–145.

Chrousos GP. 1995. The hypothalamic-pituitary-adrenal axis and immune-related inflammation. *N Engl J Med.* 332:1351–1363.

Cohen H, Benjamin J, Geva AB, et al. 2000. Autonomic dysregulation in panic disorder and in post-traumatic stress disorder: application of power spectrum analysis of heart rate variability at rest and in response to recollection of trauma or panic attacks. *Psychiatry Res.* 96:1–13.

Comings DE, Comings BG, Muhleman D, et al. 1991. The dopamine D2 receptor locus as a modifying gene in neuropsychiatric disorders. *JAMA.* 266:1793–1800.

Comings DE, Muhleman D, Gysin R. 1996. Dopamine D2 receptor (DRD2) gene and susceptibility to posttraumatic stress disorder: a study and replication. *Biological Psychiatry.* 40:368–372.

Crusto CA, Whitson ML, Walling SM, et al. 2010. Posttraumatic stress among young urban children exposed to family violence and other potentially traumatic events. *J Trauma Stress.* 23:716–724.

Davidson J, Smith R, Kudler H. 1989. Familial psychiatric illness in chronic posttraumatic stress disorder. *Comprehensive Psychiatry.* 30:339–345.

Davidson J, Swartz M, Storck M, et al. 1985. A diagnostic and family study of posttraumatic stress disorder. *Am J Psychiatry.* 142:90–93.

De Kloet ER, Reul JM. 1987. Feedback action and tonic influence of glucocorticoids on brain function: a concept arising from the heterogeneity of brain receptor systems. *Psychoneuroendrocrinology.* 12:83–105.

Delahanty DL, Dougall AL, Craig KJ, et al. 1997. Chronic stress and natural killer cell activity after exposure to traumatic death. *Psychosomatic Med.* 59:467–476.

Dougall AL, Baum A. 2004. Psychoneuroimmunology and trauma. In: Schnurr PP, Green BL, editors. *Trauma and Health: Physical Health Consequences of Exposure to Extreme Stress*. Washington, DC: American Psychological Association: 129–155.

Dragan W, Oniszczenko W. 2009. The association between dopamine D4 receptor exon III polymorphism and intensity of PTSD symptoms among flood survivors. *Anxiety, Stress, & Coping*. 22:483–495.

Drury SS, Theall KP, Keats BJB, Scheeringa M. 2009. The role of the dopamine transporter (DAT) in the development of PTSD in preschool children. *Journal of Traumatic Stress*. 22:534–539.

Ehlers A, Clark DM. 2000. A cognitive model of posttraumatic stress disorder. *Behav Res Therapy*. 38:319–345.

Ehlers A, Clark DM, Hackmann A, et al. 2005. Cognitive therapy for post-traumatic stress disorder: development and evaluation. *Behav Res Ther*. 43:413–431.

Eisen SA, True WR, Goldberg J, et al. 1987. The Vietnam Era Twin (VET) registry: method of construction. *Acta Geneticae Medical ET Gemellologiae/Twin Research*. 36:61–66.

Epstein S. 1991. The self-concept, the traumatic neurosis, and the structure of personality. In: Ozer D, Healy JM, Jr, Stewart AJ, editors. *Perspectives on personality*. Vol. 3, Part A. London: Jessica Kingsley: 63–98.

Foa EB, Kozak MJ. 1985. Treatment of anxiety disorders: implications for psychopathology. In: Tuma AH, Maser JD, editors. *Anxiety and the anxiety disorders*. Hillsdale, NJ: Erlbaum: 421–452.

Foa EB, Kozak MJ. 1986. Emotional processing of fear: exposure to corrective information. *Psychol Bull*. 99:20–35.

Foa EB, Feske U, Murdock TB, et al. 1991. Processing of threat-related information in rape victims. *J Abnorm Psychol*. 100:156–162.

Freeman T, Roca V, Guggenheim F, et al. 2005. Neuropsychiatric associations of Apolipoprotein E alleles in subjects with combat-related posttraumatic stress disorder. *J Neuropsychiatry Clin Neurosci*. 17:541–543.

Friedman MJ. 1997. Posttraumatic stress disorder. *J Clin Psychiatry*. 58(Suppl 9):33–36.

Friedman MJ, McEwen BS. 2004. Posttraumatic stress disorder: allostatic load and medical illness. In: Schnurr PP, Green BL, editors. *Trauma and health: physical health consequences of exposure to extreme stress.* Washington, DC: American Psychological Association, 157–188.

Friedman MJ, Karam EG. 2009. Posttraumatic stress disorder. In: Andrews G, Charney DS, Sirovatka PJ, Regier DA, editors. *Stress-induced and fear circuitry disorders. Advancing the research agenda for DSM-V.* Arlington, VA: American Psychiatric Association, 3–29.

Gelernter J, Southwick S, Goodson S, et al. 1999. No association between D2 dopamine receptor (DRD2) "A" system alleles, or DRD2 haplotypes, and posttraumatic stress disorder. *Biological Psychiatry.* 45:620–625.

Gerardi RJ, Keane TH, Cahoon BJ, Klauminzer GW. 1994. An in vivo assessment of physiological arousal in posttraumatic stress disorder. *J Abn Psychol.* 103:825–827.

Gilbertson MW, Gurvits TV, Lasko NB, et al. 2006. Neurocognitive function in monozygotic twins discordant for combat exposure: relationship to posttraumatic stress disorder. *J Abnormal Psychology.* 115:484–495.

Gilbertson MW, McFarlane AC, Weathers FW, et al. 2010. Is trauma a causal agent of psychopathologic symptoms in posttraumatic stress disorder? Findings from identical twins discordant for combat exposure. *J Clin Psychiatry.* 71:1324–1330.

Gilbertson MW, Shenton ME, Ciszewski A, et al. 2002. Smaller hippocampal volume predicts pathologic vulnerability to psychological trauma. *Nat Neurosci.* 5:1242–1247.

Gill JM, Szanton SL, Page GG. 2005. Biological underpinnings of health alterations in women with PTSD: a sex disparity. *Biol Res Nurs.* 7:44–54.

Gill J, Vythilingam M, Page GG. 2008. Low cortisol, high DHEA, and high levels of stimulated TNF? *J Trauma Stress.* 21:530–539.

Gotovac K, Vidovic A, Vukusic H, et al. 2010. Natural killer cell cytotoxicity and lymphocyte perforin expression in veterans with posttraumatic stress disorder. *Prog Neuropsychopharmacol Biol Psychiatry.* 34:597–604.

Grabe H, Spitzer C, Schwahn C, et al. 2009. Serotonin transporter gene (SLC6A4) promoter polymorphisms and the susceptibility to posttraumatic stress disorder in the general population. *Am J Psychiatry.* 166:926–933.

Graham-Bermann SA, Gruber G, Howell KH, Girz L. 2009. Factors discriminating among profiles of resilience and psychopathology in children exposed to intimate partner violence (IPV). *Child Abuse.* 33:648–660.

Gurvits TV, Metzger LJ, Lasko NB, et al. 2006. Subtle neurologic compromise as a vulnerability factor for combat-related posttraumatic stress disorder. *Arch Gen Psychiatry.* 63:571–576.

Gutner CA, Pineles SL, Griffin MG, et al. 2010. Physiological predictors of posttraumatic stress disorder. *J Traumatic Stress.* 23:775–784.

Hales RE, Yudofsky SC, Gabbard GO, editors. 2008. *Textbook of Psychiatry.* 5th edition. Arlington, VA: American Psychiatric Publishing Inc.

Hariri A, Mattay V, Tessitore A, et al. 2002. Serotonin transporter genetic variation and the response of the human amygdala. *Science.* 297:400–403.

Hauer D, Weis F, Papassotiropoulos A, et al. 2011. Relationship of a common polymorphism of the glucocorticoid receptor gene to traumatic memories and posttraumatic stress disorder in patients after intensive care therapy. *Critical Care Medicine.* 39:643–650.

Hoge CW, Auchterlonie JL, Milliken CS. 2006. Mental health problems, use of mental health services, and attrition from military service after returning from deployment to Iraq or Afghanistan. *Journal of the American Medical Association.* 295:1023–1032.

Horowitz MJ. 1986. *Stress response syndromes.* 2nd edition. Northvale, NJ: Aronson.

Huertas E, Ponce G, Koeneke MA, et al. 2010. The D2 dopamine receptor gene variant C957T affects human fear conditioning and aversive priming. *Genes, Brain and Behavior.* 9:103–109.

Huppert JD, Foa EB, McNally RJ, Cahill SP. 2009. In: Andrews G, Charney DS, Sirovatka PJ, Regier DA, editors. *Stress-induced and fear circuitry disorders. Advancing the research agenda for DSM-V.* Arlington, VA: American Psychiatric Association: 175–193.

Inoue-Sakurai C, Maruyama S, Morimoto K. 2000. Posttraumatic stress and lifestyles are associated with natural killer cell activity in victims of the Hanshin-Awaji earthquake in Japan. *Prev Med.* 31:467–473.

Ironson G, Wynings C, Schneiderman N, et al. 1997. Posttraumatic stress symptoms, intrusive thoughts, loss, and immune function after Hurricane Andrew. *Psychosom Med.* 59:128–141.

Jacobsen LK, Southwick SM, Kosten TR. 2001. Substance use disorders in patients with posttraumatic stress disorder: a review of the literature. *Am J Psychiatry.* 158:1184–1190.

Jang KL, Stein MB, Taylor S, et al. 2003. Exposure to traumatic events and experiences: aetiological relationships with personality function. *Psychiatry Research.* 120:61–69.

Jonas S, Bebbington P, McManus S, et al. 2011. Sexual abuse and psychiatric disorder in England: results from the 2007 Adult Psychiatric Morbidity Survey. *Psychol Med.* 41:709–719.

Karlin BE, Ruzek JI, Chard KM, et al. 2010. Dissemination of evidence-based psychological treatments for posttraumatic stress disorder in the Veterans Health Administration. *J Traumatic Stress.* 23:663–673.

Kasai K, Yamasue H, Gilbertson MW, et al. 2008. Evidence for acquired pregenual anterior cingulate gray matter loss from a twin study of combat-related post-traumatic stress disorder. *Biological Psychiatry.* 63:550–556.

Kaufman J, Aikins D, Krystal J. 2004. Neuroimaging studies in PTSD, In: Wilson JP, Keane TM, editors. *Assessing psychological trauma and PTSD.* 2nd edition. New York: Guilford: 389–418.

Kawamura N, Kim Y, Asukai N. 2001. Suppression of cellular immunity in men with a past history of posttraumatic stress disorder. *Am J Psychiatry.* 158:484–486.

Keane TM, Kolb LC, Kaloupek DG, et al. 1998. Utility of psychophysiological measurement in the diagnosis of posttraumatic stress disorder: results from a Department of Veterans Affairs cooperative study. *J Consult Clin Psychol.* 66:914–923.

Keane TM, Zimering RT, Caddell JM. 1985. A behavioral formulation of posttraumatic stress disorder. *Behavior Therapist.* 8:9–12.

Kilpatrick DG, Veronen LJ, Best CL. 1985. Factors predicting psychological distress among rape victims. In: Figley CR, editors. *Trauma and its wake.* New York: Brunner/Mazel, 113–141.

Kilpatrick DG, Koenen KC, Ruggiero KJ, et al. 2007. The serotonin transporter genotype and social support and moderation of posttraumatic stress disorder and depression in hurricane-exposed adults. *Am J Psychiatry.* 164:1693–1699.

Kimble MO, Kaufman ML, Leonard LL, et al. 2002. Sentence completion test in combat veterans with and without PTSD: preliminary findings. *Psychiatry Res.* 113:303–307.

Kimerling R. 2004. An investigation of sex differences in non-psychiatric morbidity associated with posttraumatic stress disorder. *J Am Med Womens Assoc.* 59:43–47.

Klasen F, Oettingen G, Daniels J, et al. 2010. Posttraumatic resilience in former Ugandan child soldiers. *Child Dev.* 81:1096–1113.

Kleim B, Wilhelm FH, Glucksman E, Ehlers A. 2010. Sex differences in heart rate responses to script-driven imagery soon after trauma and risk of posttraumatic stress disorder. *Psychosomatic Med.* 72:917–924.

Koenen KC, Aiello AE, Bakshis E, et al. 2009. Modification of the association between serotonin transporter genotype and risk of posttraumatic stress disorder in adults by county-level social environment. *Am J Epidemiol.* 169:704–711.

Koenen KC, Amstadter AB, Ruggiero KJ, et al. 2009. RGS2 and generalized anxiety disorder in an epidemiologic sample of hurricane-exposed adults. *Depression and Anxiety.* 26:309–315.

Koenen KC, Fu QJ, Ertel K, et al. 2008. Common genetic liability to major depression and posttraumatic stress disorder in men. *J Affect Disord.* 105:109–115.

Koenen KC, Harley R, Lyons MJ, et al. 2002. A twin registry study of familial and individual risk factors for trauma exposure and posttraumatic stress disorder. *J Nerv Ment Dis.* 190:209–218.

Koenen KC, Hitsman B, Lyons MJ, et al. 2005. A twin registry study of the relationship between posttraumatic stress disorder and nicotine dependence in men. *Arch Gen Psychiatry.* 62:1258–1265.

Koenen KC, Lyons MJ, Goldberg J, et al. 2003 Jun. A high risk twin study of combat-related PTSD comorbidity. *Twin Research.* 6:218–226.

Koenen KC, Saxe G, Purcell S, et al. 2005. Polymorphisms in FKBP5 are associated with peritraumatic dissociation in medically injured children. *Molecular Psychiatry.* 10:1058–1061.

Kolassa I, Ertl V, Eckart C, et al. 2010. Association study of trauma load and SLC6A4 promoter polymorphism in posttraumatic stress disorder: evidence from survivors of the Rwandan genocide. *J Clin Psychiatry.* 71:543–547.

Kolassa I, Kolassa S, Ertl V, et al. 2010. The risk of posttraumatic stress disorder after trauma depends on traumatic load and the catechol-O-methyltransferase Val158Met polymorphism. *Biological Psychiatry.* 67:304–308.

Kolb LC. 1989. Heterogeneity of PTSD (letter). *Am J Psychiatry.* 146:811–812.

Lader M. 1974. The peripheral and central role of the catecholamines in the mechanisms of anxiety. *Int Pharmacopsychiatry.* 9:125–137.

Lalor K, McElvaney R. 2010. Child sexual abuse, links to later sexual exploitation/high-risk sexual behavior, and prevention/treatment programs. *Trauma Violence Abuse.* 11:159–177.

Lappalainen K, Kranzler H, Malison R, et al. 2002 Sep. A functional neuropeptide Y *Leu7Pro* polymorphism associated with alcohol dependence in a large population sample from the United States. *Arch Gen Psychiatry.* 59:825–831.

Laudenslager ML, Aasal R, Adler L, et al. 1998. Elevated cytotoxicity in combat veterans with long-term post-traumatic stress disorder: preliminary observations. *Brain Behav Immun.* 12:74–79.

Lawford BR, Young RY, Noble EP, et al. 2006. The D2 dopamine receptor (DRD2) gene is associated with comorbid depression, anxiety and social dysfunction in untreated veterans with post-traumatic stress disorder. *European Psychiatry.* 21:180–185.

Lee H, Kang R, Lim W, et al. 2006. No association between the brain-derived neurotrophic factor gene Val66Met polymorphism and post-traumatic stress disorder. *Stress and Health.* 22:115–119.

Lee H, Kwak S, Maik J, et al. 2007. Association between serotonin 2A receptor gene polymorphism and posttraumatic stress disorder. *Psychiatry Investig.* 4:104–108.

Lee H, Lee M, Kang R, et al. 2005. Influence of the serotonin transporter promoter gene polymorphism on susceptibility to posttraumatic stress disorder. *Depression and Anxiety.* 21:135–139.

Lesch KP, Bengel D, Heils A, et al. 1996. Association of anxiety-related traits with a polymorphism in the serotonin transporter gene regulatory region. *Science.* 274:1527–1531.

Lu A, Ogdie M, Jarvelin M, et al. 2008. Association of the cannabinoid receptor gene (CNR1) and ADHD and post-traumatic stress disorder. *Am J Med Genet B Neuropsychiatr Genet.* 147B:1488–1494.

Lyons MJ, Goldberg J, Eisen SA, et al. 1993. Do genes influence exposure to trauma? A twin study of combat. *Am J Medical Genetics (Neuropsychiatric Genetics).* 48:22–27.

Maes M, Lin A, Bonaccorso S, et al. 1998. Increased 24-hour urinary cortisol excretion in patients with post-traumatic stress disorder and patients with major depression, but not in patients with fibromyalgia. *Acta Psychiatr Scand.* 98:328–335.

Maes M, Lin AH, Delmeire L, et al. 1999. Elevated serum interleukin-6 (IL-6) and IL-6 receptor concentrations in posttraumatic stress disorder following accidental man-made traumatic events. *Biol Psychiatry.* 45:833–839.

Maikovich AK, Koenen KC, Jaffee SR. 2009. Posttraumatic stress symptoms and trajectories in child sexual abuse victims: an analysis of sex differences using the National Survey of Child and Adolescent Well-being. *J Abnorm Child Psychol.* 37:727–737.

Margolin G, Gordis EB. 2000. The effects of family and community violence on children. *Ann Rev Psychol.* 51:445–479.

Margolin G, Vickerman KA. 2007. Post-traumatic stress in children and adolescents exposed to family violence: overview and issues. *Prof Psychol Res Pr.* 38:613–619.

Margolin G, Vickerman KA, Oliver PH, Gordis EB. 2010. Violence exposure in multiple interpersonal domains: cumulative and differential effects. *J Adolesc Health.* 47:198–205.

Mason JW, Giller EL, Kosten TR, Harkness L. 1988. Elevation of urinary norepinephrine/cortisol ratio in posttraumatic stress disorder. *J Nerv Mental Dis.* 176:498–502.

May FS, Chen QC, Gilbertson MW, et al. 2004. Cavum septum pellucidum in monozygotic twins discordant for combat exposure: relationship to posttraumatic stress disorder. *Biol Psychiatry.* 55:656–658.

Meewisse ML, Reitsma JB, de Vries GJ, et al. 2007. Cortisol and post-traumatic stress disorder in adults. Systematic review and meta-analysis. *Br J Psychiatry.* 191:387–392.

Mellman TA, Alim T, Brown DD, et al. 2009. Serotonin polymorphisms and posttraumatic stress disorder in a trauma exposed African American population. *Depression and Anxiety.* 26:993–997.

Meredith LS, Eisenman DP, Green BL, et al. 2009. System factors affect the recognition and management of posttraumatic stress disorder by primary care clinicians. *Medical Care.* 47:686–694.

McDonald R, Jouriles EN, Ramisetty-Mikler S, et al. 2006. Estimating the number of American children living in partner-violent families. *J Fam Psychol.* 20:137–142.

McFarlane AC. 2010. The long-term costs of traumatic stress: intertwined physical and psychological consequences. *World Psychiatry.* 29:3–10.

McNally RJ. 1998. Experimental approaches to cognitive abnormality in posttraumatic stress disorder. *Clin Psychol Rev.* 18:971–982.

Miller RJ, Sutherland AG, Hutchison JD, Alexander DA. 2001. C-reactive protein and interleukin 6 receptor in post-traumatic stress disorder: a pilot study. *Cytokine.* 13:253–255.

Mimiaga MJ, Noonan E, Donnell D, et al. 2009. Childhood sexual abuse is highly associated with HIV risk-taking behavior and infection among MSM in the EXPLORE Study. *J Acquir Immune Defic Syndr.* 51:340–348.

Mosnaim AD, Wolf ME, Maturana P, et al. 1993. In vitro studies of natural killer cell activity in post traumatic stress disorder patients. Response to methionine-enkephalin challenge. *Immunopharmacology.* 25:107–116.

Mueser KT, Taub J. 2008. Trauma and PTSD among adolescents with severe emotional disorders involved in multiple service systems. *Psychiatric Services.* 59:627–634.

Munafo MR, Yalcin B, Willis-Owen SA, Flint J. 2008. Association of the dopamine D4 receptor (DRD4) gene and approach-related personality traits: Meta-analysis and new data. *Biological Psychiatry.* 63:197–206.

Mustapic M, Pivac N, Kozaric-Kovacic D, et al. 2007. Dopamine beta-hydroxylase (DBH) activity and –1021C/T polymorphism of DBH gene in combat-related post-traumatic stress disorder. *Am J Med Gen Part B.* 144B:1087–1089.

Nakamura M, Ueno S, Sano A, Tanabe H. 2000. The human serotonin transporter gene linked polymorphism (5-HTTLPR) shows ten novel allelic variants. *Molecular Psychiatry.* 5:32–38.

Nelson EC, Agrawal A, Pergadia ML, et al. 2009. Association of childhood trauma exposure and GABRA2 polymorphisms with risk of posttraumatic stress disorder in adults. *Molecular Psychiatry.* 14:234–238.

Neylan TC, Sun B, Rempel H, et al. 2010. Suppressed monocyte gene expression profile in men versus women with PTSD. *Brain Behav Immun.* 25:524–531.

Pitman RK, Gilbertson MW, Gurvits TV, et al. 2006. Clarifying the origin of biological abnormalities in PTSD through the study of identical twins discordant for combat exposure. *Ann NY Acad Sci.* 1071:242–254.

Rauch SL, Drevets WC. 2009. Neuroimaging and neuroanatomy of stress-induced and fear circuitry disorders. In: Andrews G, Charney DS, Sirovatka PJ, Regier DA, editors. *Stress-induced and fear circuitry disorders. Advancing the research agenda for DSM-V.* Arlington, VA: American Psychiatric Association: 215–254.

Ressler K, Mercer K, Bradley B, et al. 2011. Post-traumatic stress disorder is associated with PACAP and the PAC1 receptor. *Nature.* 470:492–497.

Robinson BL, Shergill SS. 2011. Imaging in posttraumatic stress disorder. *Curr Opin Psychiatry.* 24:29–33.

Rohleder N, Karl A. 2006. Role of endocrine and inflammatory alterations in comorbid somatic diseases of post-traumatic stress disorder. *Minerva Endocrinol.* 31:273–288.

Rubin DC, Bernsten D, Johansen MK. 2008. A memory based model of posttraumatic stress disorder: evaluating basic assumptions underlying the PTSD diagnosis. *Psychol Rev.* 115:985–1011.

Sack WH, Clarke GN, Seeley J. 1995. Posttraumatic stress disorder across two generations of Cambodian refugees. *J Am Acad Child Adolesc Psychiatry.* 34:1160–1166.

Sayin A, Kucukyildirim S, Skar R, et al. 2010. A prospective study of serotonin transporter gene promoter (5-HTT gene linked polymorphic region) and intron 2 (variable number of tandem repeats) polymorphisms as predictors of trauma response to mild physical injury. *DNA and Cell Biology.* 29:71–77.

Schmidt U, Hosboer F, Rein T. 2011. Epigenetic aspects of posttraumatic stress disorder. *Dis Markers.* 30:77–87.

Schnurr PP, Green BL. 2004. Understanding relationships among trauma, post-traumatic stress disorder, and health outcomes. *Advances.* 20:18–29.

Segman RH, Shefi N, Goltser-Dubner T, et al. 2005. Peripheral blood mononuclear cell gene expression profiles identify emergent post-traumatic stress disorder among trauma survivors. *Molecular Psychiatry.* 10:500–513.

Segman RH, Cooper-Kazaz, Macciardi F, et al. 2002. Association between the dopamine transporter gene and posttraumatic stress disorder. *Molecular Psychiatry.* 7:903–907.

Skre I, Onstad S, Torgersen S, et al. 1993. A twin study of DSM-III-R anxiety disorders. *Acta Psychiatr Scan.* 88:85–92.

Spivak B, Shohat B, Mester R, et al. 1997. Elevated levels of serum interleukin-1 beta in combat-related posttraumatic stress disorder. *Biol Psychiatry.* 12:345–348.

Spoont MR, Murdoch M, Hodges J, Nugent S. 2010. Treatment receipt by veterans after a PTSD diagnosis in PTSD, mental health, or general medical clinics. *Psychiatric Services.* 61:58–63.

Stein MB, Jang KL, Taylor S, et al. 2002. Genetic and environmental influences on trauma exposure and posttraumatic stress disorder symptoms: a twin study. *Am J Psychiatry.* 159:1675–1681.

Tang Y, Li W, Mercer K, Bradley B, et al. 2010. Genotype-controlled analysis of serum dopamine β-hydroxylase activity in civilian post-traumatic stress disorder. *Progress in Neuro-Psychopharmacology & Biological Psychiatry.* 34:1396–1401.

Thakur GA, Joober R, Brunet A. 2009. Development and persistence of posttraumatic stress disorder and the 5-HTTLPR polymorphism. *Journal of Traumatic Stress.* 22:240–243.

True WR, Rice J, Eisen SA, et al. 1993. A twin study of genetic and environmental contributions to liability for posttraumatic stress symptoms. *Arch Gen Psychiatry.* 50:257–264.

Tucker P, Ruwe WD, Masters B, et al. 2004. Neuroimmune and cortisol changes in selective serotonin reuptake inhibitor and placebo treatment of chronic posttraumatic stress disorder. *Biol Psychiatry.* 56:121–128.

Uddin M, Aiello AE, Wildman DE, et al. 2010. Epigenetic and immune function profiles associated with posttraumatic stress disorder. *Proc Natl Acad Sci USA.* 107:9470–9475.

Valente N, Vallada H, Cordiero Q, et al. 2011. Candidate-gene approach in posttraumatic stress disorder after urban violence: association studies of the genes encoding serotonin transporter, dopamine transporter, and BDNF. *J Mol Neurosci* 44:59–67.

Valente N, Vallada H, Cordiero Q, et al. 2011. Catechol-O-methyltransferase (COMT) val158met polymorphism as a risk factor for PTSD after urban violence. *J Mol Neurosci.* 43:516–523.

Vidovic A, Vilibic M, Sabioncello A, et al. 2007. Circulating lymphocyte subsets, natural killer cell cytotoxicity, and components of hypothalamic-pituitary-adrenal axis in

Croatian War veterans with posttraumatic stress disorder: cross-sectional study. *Croat Med J.* 48:198–206.

Voisey J, Swagell CD, Hughes IP, et al. 2009. The DRD2 gene 957C>T polymorphism is associated with posttraumatic stress disorder in war veterans. *Depression and Anxiety.* 26:28–33.

Voisey J, Swagell CD, Hughes IP, et al. 2010. A polymorphism in the dysbindin gene (DTNBP1) associated with multiple psychiatric disorders including schizophrenia. *Behavioral and Brain Functions.* 6:41.

Watson IP, Muller HK, Jones IH, Bradley AJ. 1993. Cell-mediated immunity in combat veterans with post-traumatic stress disorder. *Med J Aust.* 159:513–516.

Wilson SN, van der Kolk B, Burbridge J, et al. 1999. Phenotype of blood lymphocytes in PTSD suggests chronic immune activation. *Psychosomatics.* 40:222–225.

Woods SJ, Wineman NM, Page GG, et al. 2005. Predicting immune status in women from PTSD and childhood and adult violence. *ANS Adv Nurs Sci.* 28:306–319.

Yehuda R. 2000. Biology of posttraumatic stress disorder. *J Clin Psychiatry.* 61(Suppl 7):14–21.

Yehuda R, Bierer LM. 2009. The relevance of epigenetics to PTSD: implications for the DSM-V. *J Trauma Stress.* 22:427–434.

Yehuda R, Boisoneau D, Mason JW, et al. 1993. Glucocorticoid receptor number and cortisol excretion in mood, anxiety, and psychotic disorders. *Biol Psychiatry.* 34:18–25.

Yehuda R, Cai G, Golier JA, et al. 2009. Gene expression patterns associated with posttraumatic stress disorder following exposure to the World Trade Center attacks. *Biological Psychiatry.* 66:708–711.

Yehuda R, Engel SM, Brand SR, et al. 2005. Transgenerational effects of posttraumatic stress disorder in babies of mothers exposed to the World Trade Center attacks during pregnancy. *Journal of Clinical Endocrinology & Metabolism.* 90:4115–4118.

Yehuda R, Halligan SL, Bierer LM. 2001. Relationship of parental trauma exposure and PTSD to PTSD, depressive and anxiety disorders in offspring. *Journal of Psychiatric Research.* 35:261–270.

Yehuda R, Halligan SL, Bierer LM. 2002. Cortisol levels in adult offspring of Holocaust survivors: relation to PTSD symptom severity in the parent and child. *Psychoneuroendocrinology.* 27:171–180.

Yehuda R, Schmeidler J, Giller EL, et al. 1998. Relationship between posttraumatic stress disorder characteristics of Holocaust survivors and their adult offspring. *Am J Psychiatry.* 155:841–843.

Xian H, Chantarujikapong SI, Scherrer JF, et al. 2000. Genetic and environmental influences on posttraumatic stress disorder, alcohol and drug dependence in twin pairs. *Alcohol and Drug Dependence.* 61:95–102.

Xie P, Kranzler HB, Poling J, et al. 2009. Interactive effect of stressful life events and the serotonin transporter 5-HTTLPR genotype on posttraumatic stress disorder diagnosis in 2 independent populations. *Arch Gen Psychiatry.* 66:1201–1209.

Xie P, Kranzler H, Poling J, et al. 2010. Interaction of FKBP5 with childhood adversity on risk for post-traumatic stress disorder. *Neuropsychopharmacology.* 35:1684–1692.

Young RM, Lawford BR, Noble EP, et al. 2002. Harmful drinking in military veterans with post-traumatic stress disorder: association with the D2 dopamine receptor A1 allele. *Alcohol & Alcoholism.* 37:451–456.

Zhang H, Ozbay F, Lappalainen J, et al. 2006. Brain derived neurotrophic factor gene (*BDNF*) variants and Alzheimer's Disease, affective disorders, posttraumatic stress disorder, schizophrenia and substance dependence. *Am J Med Genet B Neuropsychiatr Genet.* 141B:387–393.

Zieker J, Zieker D, Jatzko A, et al. 2007. Differential gene expression in peripheral blood of patients suffering from post-traumatic stress disorder. *Molecular Psychiatry.* 12:116–118.

2

The Epidemiology of Post-Traumatic Stress Disorder

Steven S. Coughlin, Ph.D.

Epidemiologic studies have provided important insights about the incidence, prevalence, and chronicity of post-traumatic stress disorder (PTSD) in the general population; in population subgroups defined by age, gender, race, or ethnicity; and in high-risk populations such as combat veterans, military personnel, and women and men who are victims of rape or other violent crimes (Breslau and Davis 1992; Kang et al. 2009; Hoge et al. 2004; Kimerling et al. 2010). The lifetime prevalence of PTSD has been estimated to be about 6.4–9% among persons in the U.S. (Kennedy et al. 2007; Kessler et al. 2005a; Pietrzak et al. 2010). International variation in PTSD rates has been reported in studies of persons injured in severe motor vehicle accidents (Harvey and Bryant 1998; Murray et al. 2002; Schnyder et al. 2001). About half of persons who develop PTSD eventually recover from their illness, although many do not (Breslau and Davis 1992; Yehuda 2000). As discussed in other chapters in this book, co-occurring health conditions may partly account for why some persons are less apt to recover from PTSD or have a more severe course of illness.

MEASUREMENT OF PTSD IN POPULATION SURVEYS

Self-report measures are commonly used in population surveys to estimate the prevalence of PTSD. The PTSD Checklist (PCL) is a commonly used instrument for assessing PTSD symptoms based upon self-reported information (Weathers et al. 1993; Terhakopian et al. 2008). The PCL is a 17-item questionnaire based on the criteria provided in the Diagnostic and Statistical

Manual of Mental disorders, fourth edition (DSM-IV). More than one version of PCL exists including a version intended for military personnel (PCL-M) and one for civilians exposed to traumatic experiences (PCL-C). Respondents rate PCL items on a 5-point Likert-type scale to indicate the degree to which they have had each of 17 PTSD symptoms during the past month. The most commonly used approach for scoring involves summing the response from the 17 PCL items to obtain a score ranging from 17 to 85 and then selecting a cutoff (for example, considering respondents with a score of 50 or higher to have PTSD). Another approach for scoring relies on DSM-IV symptom criteria for PTSD. Persons who report at least one reexperiencing symptom, three avoidance symptoms, and two hyperarousal symptoms at the moderate level of distress or higher are considered to have PTSD (Terhakopian et al. 2008). These two approaches for PCL scoring can be combined (Hoge et al. 2004). The PCL has been shown to have good test-retest reliability and validity when comparisons have been made with structured clinical diagnostic interviews. Nevertheless, the optimal cutoff score for identifying persons with PTSD varies according to the true population prevalence of PTSD (Weathers et al. 1993; Terhakopian et al. 2008).

Changes in definitions of PTSD over time, beginning with DSM-III in 1980 and extending to DSM-IV-TR and beyond, create challenges for comparing results across epidemiologic studies conducted at different times. For example, assessments of PTSD prevalence rates based upon DSM-IV criteria tend to be lower than those based upon DSM-III-R criteria (Breslau 2002; Norris and Slone 2007). However, refinements in diagnostic criteria for PTSD help differentiate PTSD from other anxiety and mood disorders (for example, major depression) and likely improve the specificity of diagnoses.

Partial or Subthreshold PTSD

Persons exposed to trauma may experience some PTSD symptoms but not enough to make the full diagnosis. Such persons have been considered to have partial or subthreshold PTSD in some studies of veteran and civilian populations (Kulka et al. 1990; Stein et al. 1997; Laugharne et al. 2010; Marshall et al. 2001; Pietrzak et al. 2010). Cases of partial PTSD have insufficient symptoms or less than the three required symptom groups to meet criteria for full PTSD (Carlier and Gersons 1995). Stein et al. (1997) examined full and partial PTSD in a random sample of 1,002 persons from a community survey conducted in a Midwestern Canadian city. The researchers determined current prevalence rates of full PTSD (which met all DSM-IV criteria) and partial PTSD, which met fewer than the required number of DSM-IV criterion C symptoms (avoidance/numbing) or criterion D symptoms (increased arousal). The estimated prevalence of full PTSD was 2.7% for women and 1.2% for men. The prevalence of partial PTSD was 3.4% for women and 0.3% for men (Stein et al. 1997). The authors noted that many traumatized persons may suffer from a subsyndromal form of PTSD which is associated with clinically significant levels of functional impairment. Studies have shown that people with partial PTSD experience less interference with work than people with full PTSD. However, studies of community samples and disaster survivors have shown that persons with partial PTSD experience greater impairment and more suicidal ideation than persons without partial or full PTSD (Carlier and Gersons 1995; Cukor et al. 2010; Marshall et al. 2001). Longitudinal studies are needed to determine whether cases of partial or subthreshold PTSD represent persons who never met criteria for full PTSD, or whether they represent persons who previously had full PTSD but are currently in partial remission.

EPIDEMIOLOGY OF PTSD IN MILITARY AND VETERAN POPULATIONS

Epidemiologic studies have shown that may combat veterans in the United States and other countries suffer from PTSD, although estimates vary according to era of military service, intensity of combat exposures, and other factors (Kulka and Schlenger 1990; Friedman et al. 1994; Dohrenwend et al. 2006; Fear et al. 2010). The extensive research on PTSD among U.S. veterans who served in the Vietnam War includes analyses of data from the Vietnam Experience Study and the National Vietnam Veterans Readjustment Study (Kulka and Schlenger 1990; Boscarino 2004). In the National Vietnam Veterans Readjustment Study, an estimated 15.2% of male and 8.5% of female Vietnam theater veterans met criteria for current PTSD (Kulka and Schlenger 1990; Schlenger et al. 1992). Those with high levels of war-zone exposure had higher rates of current PTSD (35.8% of men and 17.5% of women). The rates of lifetime PTSD among male and female Vietnam theater veterans were 30.9% and 26.9%, respectively. Another study of the lifetime prevalence of PTSD in male Vietnam War veterans found a 30% prevalence rate compared with 5% among men in the general population (Koenen et al. 2002).

Among U.S. veterans who served in the Gulf War (1990–1991), studies have generally found lower PTSD rates than in Vietnam War veterans or recent veterans who served in Operation Enduring Freedom and Operation Iraqi Freedom, which is consistent with the shorter duration of the conflict. Estimates of the rate of PTSD among 1990–1991 Gulf War veterans have ranged from 1.9% to 15.2% (Holmes et al. 1998; Proctor et al. 1998; Wolfe et al. 1999; Steele 2000; Barrett et al. 2002; Blanchard et al. 2006; Fiedler et al. 2006; Toomey et al. 2007; Kang et al. 2003, 2009). Rates have varied according to approaches used to measure PTSD (for example, structured clinical interview versus PCL, or other self-reported questionnaires) and time since return from deployment.

Estimates of PTSD among U.S. Army and Marine Corps personnel who served in Operation Enduring Freedom and Operation Iraqi Freedom have ranged from 10% to 18% (Hoge et al. 2004, 2006, 2007; Grieger et al. 2006; Erbes et al. 2007; Seal et al. 2007; Schell and Marshall 2008; Vasterling et al. 2008, 2010; Vogt et al. 2011a; Vogt et al. 2011b). Hoge et al. (2004) surveyed members of four U.S. combat infantry units either before their deployment to Iraq (n = 2,530) or three to four months after their return from combat duty in Iraq or Afghanistan (n = 3,671). In the Army study group, about 5% (120 of 2,414) had PTSD prior to deployment according to strict PCL criteria (PCL score $\geq$ 50). After deployment to Iraq, about 12.9% (114 of 881) of the Army study group had PTSD and 12.2% (99 of 811) of the Marine study group (Hoge et al. 2004). Studies conducted in 2003 and 2004 showed that military service men and women returning from deployment in Iraq were more likely to report a mental health problem than those returning from deployment in Afghanistan (Hoge et al. 2004, 2006). Smith et al. (2008) examined self-reported, new onset PTSD symptoms and diagnoses among U.S. military personnel enrolled in the Millennium Cohort Study. New onset PTSD symptoms or diagnoses were identified in 7.6% to 8.7% of deployed personnel who reported combat exposures compared with 2.3% to 3.0% of those who had not been deployed (Smith et al. 2008). The authors noted that specific combat exposures, rather than deployment itself, significantly affect the onset of PTSD symptoms. Additional analyses of data from the Millennium Cohort Study and other U.S. and United Kingdom military populations have shown that poorer mental or physical health status before combat exposure, preinjury psychological symptoms and psychiatric status, and injury severity increase the risk of PTSD symptoms or diagnosis following deployment (LeardMann et al. 2009; Rona et al. 2009; Sandweiss et al. 2011; Vogt et al. 2011b). Differences in PTSD rates observed across studies of military personnel from the United States, the United Kingdom, and other countries are likely to be due in part to variation in measures used to assess PTSD, study design, and the population sampled (Milliken et al. 2007; Ramchand et al. 2008; Smith et al. 2009; Fear et al. 2010).

Among troops exposed to combat, PTSD is more common among those suffering from a physical injury (MacGregor et al. 2009). Higher intensity of combat exposure, longer military deployments, and less time between deployments have also been associated with increased risk of PTSD (Shen et al. 2009; Vasterling et al. 2010).

Predeployment resilience training and greater unit cohesiveness are likely to protect against PTSD and other psychiatric disorders. Studies have shown that risk of PTSD is increased among persons with a younger age of entry into the military and less premilitary education (Friedman et al. 1994).

Military-related sexual trauma has also been associated with PTSD in both female and male veterans, although military sexual trauma is much more frequent among female veterans in the United States (Suris et al. 2004; Sadler et al. 2003, 2004; Kang et al. 2005; Kimerling et al. 2007, 2009; Suris and Lind 2008). In a study of 270 women veterans receiving medical or mental health treatment at the Veterans Affairs North Texas Healthcare system, Suris et al. (2004) found that women veterans were nine times more likely to have PTSD if they had a history of military sexual trauma. Kimerling et al. (2010) examined military sexual trauma among veterans who had been deployed to Operation Enduring Freedom and Operation Iraqi Freedom, using Veterans Health Administration administrative databases. Of 125,729 veterans who received primary care or mental health services, 15.1% of the women and 0.7% of the men reported military sexual trauma when screened. Military sexual trauma was positively associated with PTSD (Kimerling et al. 2010).

PTSD IN CIVILIAN POPULATIONS

In civilian populations, a wide variety of factors have been associated with higher risk of developing PTSD including rape, being physically assaulted during a crime, witnessing a homicide, and being a survivor of a natural or man-made disaster (Kennedy et al. 2007; Norris and Slone 2007). Epidemiologic studies of PTSD in communities and diverse populations have provided important insights about the distribution and determinants of the disorder, beyond those gained from studies of relatively selected groups of patients seeking clinical treatment. Other aspects of the natural history of PTSD to which epidemiologic studies have contributed insights include delayed-onset PTSD (Horesch et al. 2010; McFarlance 2010) and the course of PTSD in children and adolescents (Green et al. 1991; Honig et al. 1993; Copeland et al. 2007). Population-based studies have also provided information about the prevalence of trauma exposure (Hidalgo and Davidson 2000).

Prevalence of Trauma in Civilian Populations

Several studies have examined the prevalence of traumatic experience in civilian populations in the U.S. and other countries (Resnick et al. 1993; Kessler et al. 1995; Hidalgo and Davidson 2000; Creamer et al. 2001; Mills 2006). Findings from these studies indicate that trauma is a frequent event. For example, Resnick et al. (1993) examined the prevalence of trauma and PTSD among 4,008 adult women. The researchers found an overall lifetime exposure to crime or non-crime-related trauma of 69%. About 12.6% of the women had been traumatized by rape, 14.3% by molestation or attempted sexual assault, 10.3% by physical assault, and 13.4% by the death of a close friend or relative by homicide (Resnick et al. 1993). In the National Comorbidity Survey, Kessler et al. (1995) found a prevalence rate of exposure to one or more traumatic events of 51.2% in women and 60.6% in men. Among persons who had been exposed to trauma, 12.5% of women and 17% of men had a history of more than three traumatic exposures in their lifetime (Kessler et al. 1995). Breslau et al. (1991) examined the prevalence of traumatic exposures in a sample of 1,007 young adults aged 21–30 years from a health maintenance organization in Detroit, Michigan. A total of 39.1% of the people in the sample had one or more traumatic experiences. The most common traumatic experiences were sudden injury or serious accident, physical assault, seeing someone seriously hurt or killed, and hearing about the sudden death of a close friend or relative (Breslau et al. 1991). Although data are sparse outside of developed countries such as the United States, large proportions of populations in many countries have been exposed to forced relocation, armed conflicts (or other violence), natural disasters such as earthquakes and typhoons, and other traumatic events (De Jong et al. 2001; Galea et al. 2005).

Prevalence and Chronicity of PTSD in Civilian Populations

The lifetime prevalence of PTSD has been estimated to be about 6.4–9% among persons in the United States (Kennedy et al. 2007; Kessler et al. 2005a; Pietrzak et al. 2010). In the National Comorbidity Survey Replication, the 12-month prevalence of PTSD was estimated to be 3.5% (Kessler et al. 2005b). In an analysis of data from wave two of the National Epidemiologic Survey of Alcohol and Related Conditions (n = 34,653), Pietrzak et al. (2010) found that the lifetime prevalence of PTSD and partial PTSD was 6.4% and 6.6%, respectively. In the United States, about 8-14% of men exposed to trauma, and about 20–31% of women exposed to trauma develop PTSD (Schnurr and Green 2004). Although about 25% of persons develop PTSD as a result of trauma overall, this percentage varies according to the severity of the traumatic event (Kessler et al. 1995; Yehuda 2000). Roughly half of persons who develop PTSD eventually recover from their illness (Breslau and Davis 1992; Yehuda 2000). The above-mentioned study by Breslau and Davis (1992) of a suburban population of young adults (n = 1,007) provided important information about the chronicity of PTSD. In their cross-sectional study, members of the health maintenance organization were interviewed using the Diagnostic Interview Schedule, revised for DSM-III-R. The analysis focused on data from 394 respondents who reported traumatic events, of whom 93 met criteria for PTSD. About 57% of persons with PTSD had chronic PTSD, defined as symptoms that persisted for one year or more. Persons with chronic PTSD (n = 53) had a higher total number of PTSD symptoms, higher rates of interpersonal numbing (detachment from others), and higher rates of overreactivity to stimuli that symbolized the stressor than persons with nonchronic PTSD. The studies found that women were at greater risk for PTSD than men, even though they were not more likely than men to be exposed to traumatic events (Breslau et al. 1991; Breslau and Davis 1992). Women comprised 83% of those with chronic PTSD lasting 1 year or more.

Risk Factors for PTSD in Civilian Populations

Epidemiologic studies have identified several risk factors for PTSD including the severity or duration of exposure to trauma. Certain violent acts including rape have been found to be more likely to result in PTSD. In the National Comorbidity Survey, Kessler et al. (1995) found that rape showed the highest conditional probability of leading to PTSD in both women and men. PTSD rates were also found to vary by type of trauma in the study by Resnick et al. (1993). Other PTSD risk factors identified in epidemiologic studies include prior history of depression or anxiety disorder, prior history of trauma including childhood abuse or neglect, having a positive family history of psychiatric illness, and younger age at time of traumatic exposure (Hidalgo and Davidson 2000). Kilpatrick et al. (2003) examined PTSD in a sample of 4,023 adolescents using a modified version of the Diagnostic Interview Schedule for DSM-III-R. The lifetime prevalence of PTSD was 10% among girls and 6% among boys. Adolescents who had suffered multiple sexual assaults were at highest risk of PTSD (Kilpatrick et al. 2003).

Race and ethnicity have not been consistently found to be associated with risk of PTSD in epidemiologic studies. The lack of consistency in studies of racial or ethnic differences in PTSD may be partly due to misdiagnosis, underdiagnosis, or uncontrolled confounding by other variables such as the severity or frequency of traumatic exposures (Lawson 2009). Roberts et al. (2011a) examined racial and ethnic differences in PTSD among 34,653 adults who had been surveyed using structured diagnostic interviews as part of the 2004–2005 wave of the National Epidemiologic Survey on Alcohol and Related Conditions. The lifetime prevalence of PTSD was highest among those of African descent (8.7%), followed by Hispanics (7%), Caucasians (7.4%), and Asians (4%). Racial and ethnic differences in exposure to trauma and treatment-seeking behaviors may partly account for the observed differences (Roberts et al. 2011b). Sexual minorities in the United States have also been reported to have higher exposures to traumatic events, beginning in childhood, and higher risk of PTSD than heterosexual persons (Roberts et al. 2011b).

Gender has also been found to be an important risk factor for PTSD. The lifetime prevalence of PTSD varies by sex with a female-to-male lifetime prevalence ratio of about 2 to 1 (Kennedy et al. 2007). The population prevalence of PTSD is about 5–6% in men and 10–12% in women (Breslau et al. 1991; Resnick et al. 1993; Kessler et al. 1995). In their analysis of data from wave two of the National Epidemiologic Survey of Alcohol and Related Conditions (n = 34,653), Pietrzak et al. (2010) found that the lifetime prevalence of PTSD and partial PTSD was higher among women (8.6% and

8.6%) than men (4.1% and 4.5%). Women have a higher risk of PTSD even though they are less frequently exposed to traumatic situations (Hidalgo and Davidson 2000). Studies have indicated that gender may moderate the associations between traumatic exposures and PTSD (Luxton et al. 2010; Dell'osso et al. 2011; Fan et al. 2011).

PTSD Following Natural or Man-Made Disasters

An increasing number of epidemiologic studies have examined PTSD among persons exposed to natural or man-made disasters (North et al. 1999, 2005; de Jong et al. 2001; Bleich et al. 2003; Galea et al. 2003; Verger et al. 2004; Galea et al. 2005; Acierno 2007; Canetti et al. 2010; DiGrande et al. 2010; Yang et al. 2010). Additional studies have examined PTSD among children and adolescents exposed to trauma (Green et al. 1991; Honig et al. 1993; Copeland et al. 2007; Yang et al. 2010). Kohn et al. (2005) interviewed 800 persons age 15 and older in Tegucigalpa, Honduras, two months after Hurricane Mitch had caused destruction in the area. The participants were selected from residential areas of high, middle, or low socioeconomic status that had suffered either high or low impact from the devastating effects of the hurricane. Respondents from high-impact residential areas were more distressed and had greater severity of PTSD symptoms (Kohn et al. 2005). Predictors of PTSD included degree of exposure based upon reported traumatic events. Among those with PTSD, women and those with a higher degree of exposure to hurricane-related traumatic events had a greater severity of PTSD on average (Kohn et al. 2005). Acierno et al. (2007) surveyed a sample of 1,452 adults 6–9 months following the 2004 Florida hurricanes. The overall prevalence of PTSD among those affected by the hurricane was 36%. Storm exposure variables, displacement, and low social support were positively associated with PTSD (Acierno et al. 2007). Studies of Hurricane Katrina survivors have also found a high prevalence of PTSD symptoms (Kishore et al. 2008; DeSalvo et al. 2007). Yang et al. (2010) examined the prevalence of PTSD among 271 adolescents who were displaced by Typhoon Morakot in Taiwan. The overall prevalence of PTSD was 25.8% among those persons affected by the typhoon. Adolescents who were female, or had a prior traumatic event, were physically injured, or had a family member in the same household who died or was seriously injured, were more likely to have PTSD (Yang et al.

2010). Amstadter et al. (2009) found a prevalence of PTSD of only 2.6% in a study of 798 persons in Vietnam who were survivors of Typhoon Xangsane.

Epidemiologic studies of PTSD among persons exposed to man-made disasters include surveys of persons exposed to terrorist acts (North et al. 1999, 2005; Galea et al. 2003; Verger et al. 2004; DiGrande et al. 2011) and civilian populations exposed to war or mass violence (Bleich et al. 2003; de Jong et al. 2001; Canetti et al. 2010). For example, Galea et al. (2003) examined the prevalence of probable PTSD in the general population of New York City in the first 6 months after the September 11, 2001, terrorist attacks. The prevalence of PTSD symptoms, which declined over time, was higher among persons who were more directly affected by the attacks. In a survey conducted 2–3 years after the September 11, 2001 terrorist attacks, DiGrande et al. (2010) found that 15.0% of 3,271 civilians who had been evacuated from the World Trade Center Towers one and two met PCL criteria for PTSD. Cross-cultural studies have demonstrated the potential for persons to develop PTSD in the aftermath of terrorist acts and other mass violence in countries around the world (de Jong et al. 2001; North et al. 2005).

SUMMARY AND CONCLUSIONS

This chapter has provided a summary of the epidemiology of PTSD in order to help provide a foundation for the chapters that follow. Although much of the available data are from studies conducted in the United States and other developed countries, results from epidemiologic studies indicate that a substantial proportion of the general population is exposed to traumatic events and that up to 9% of persons in the United States have a lifetime prevalence of PTSD. Although DSM diagnoses such as PTSD may be "culture-bound syndromes" since they originated in Western psychiatry, an increasing number of studies have examined PTSD in diverse cultures around the globe (de Jong et al. 2001; North et al. 2005; Myer et al. 2008; Martin and Kagee 2011).

While self-reported screening tools such as PCL are commonly used to assess PTSD symptoms in population surveys, information from clinical diagnostic interviews provides important information to validate self-reported information. Changes in diagnostic criteria for PTSD over time create a continuing challenge for comparing results across studies conducted in different time periods.

Key risk factors for PTSD examined in epidemiologic studies include: (1) rape and sexual assault; (2) physical assault and other acts of violence; (3) combat exposures during military service; (4) prior history of childhood abuse or neglect; (5) having a positive family history of psychiatric illness; (6) sex or gender; and (7) younger age at time of traumatic exposure. Epidemiologic studies have also shown that the duration and severity of the trauma are also related to risk of PTSD. In addition to PTSD, traumatic events increase vulnerability to several psychiatric disorders including generalized anxiety disorder, acute anxiety disorder, major depressive disorder and other mood disorders, as discussed in Chapter 3.

REFERENCES

Acierno R, Ruggiero KJ, Galea S, et al. 2007. Psychological sequelae resulting from the 2004 Florida hurricanes: implications for postdisaster intervention. *Am J Public Health.* 97(Suppl 1):S103–S108.

Amstadter AB, Acierno R, Richardson L, et al. 2009. Post-typhoon prevalence of post-traumatic stress disorder, major depressive disorder, panic disorder and generalized anxiety disorder in a Vietnamese sample. *J Trauma Stress.* 22:180–188.

Barrett DH, Doebbeling CC, Schwartz DA, et al. 2002. Posttraumatic stress disorder and self-reported physical health status among U.S. military personnel serving during the Gulf War period. A population-based study. *Psychosomatics.* 43:195–205.

Blanchard MS, Eisen SA, Alpern R, et al. 2006. Chronic multisymptom illness complex in Gulf War I veterans 10 years later. *Am J Epidemiol.* 163:66–75.

Bleich A, Gelkopf M, Solomon Z. 2003. Exposure to terrorism, stress-related mental health symptoms, and coping behaviors among a nationally representative sample in Israel. *JAMA.* 290:612–620.

Boscarino JA. 2004. Posttraumatic stress disorder and physical illness. Results from clinical and epidemiologic studies. *Ann NY Acad Sci.* 1032:141–153.

Breslau N. 2002. Epidemiologic studies of trauma, posttraumatic stress disorder, and other psychiatric disorders. *Can J Psychiatry.* 47:923–929.

Breslau N, Davis GC. 1992. Posttraumatic stress disorder in an urban population of young adults: risk factors for chronicity. *Am J Psychiatry.* 49:671–675.

Breslau N, Davis GC, Andreski P, Peterson EL. 1991. Traumatic events and posttraumatic stress disorder in an urban population of young adults. *Arch Gen Psychiatry*. 48:216–222.

Breslau N, Lucia VC, Davis GC. 2004. Partial PTSD versus full PTSD: an empirical examination of associated impairment. *Psychol Med*. 34:1205–1214.

Canetti D, Galea S, Hall BJ, et al. 2010. Exposure to prolonged socio-political conflict and the risk of PTSD and depression among Palestinians. *Psychiatry*. 73:219–231.

Carlier IVE, Gersons BPR. 1995. Partial posttraumatic stress disorder (PTSD): the issue of psychological scars and the occurrence of PTSD symptoms. *J Nerv Mental Dis*. 183:107–109.

Copeland WE, Keeler G, Angold A, Costello EJ. 2007. Traumatic events and posttraumatic stress in childhood. *Arch Gen Psychiatry*. 64:577–584.

Creamer M, Burgess PM, McFarlane AC. 2001. Post-traumatic stress disorder: findings from the Australian National Survey of Mental Health and Well-Being. *Psychological Med*. 31:1237–1247.

Cukor J, Wyka K, Jayasinghe N, Difede J. 2010. The nature and course of subthreshold PTSD. *J Anxiety Disord*. 24:918–923.

De Jong JT, Komproe IH, Van Ommeren M, et al. 2001. Lifetime events and posttraumatic stress disorder in 4 postconflict settings. *JAMA*. 286:555–562.

Dell'osso L, Carmassi C, Massimetti G, et al. 2011. Full and partial PTSD among young adult survivors 10 months after the L'Aquila 2009 earthquake: gender differences. *J Affect Disord*.131:79–83.

DeSalvo KB, Hyre AD, Ompad DC, et al. 2007. Symptoms of posttraumatic stress disorder in a New Orleans workforce following Hurricane Katrina. *J Urban Health*. 84:142–152.

DiGrande L, Neria Y, Brackbill RM, et al. 2010. Long-term posttraumatic stress symptoms among 3,271 civilian survivors of the September 11, 2001, terrorist attacks on the World Trade Center. *Am J Epidemiol*. 173:271–281.

Dohrenwend BP, Turner JB, Turse NA, et al. 2006. The psychological risks of Vietnam for U.S. veterans: a revisit with new data and methods. *Science*. 313:979–982.

Erbes C, Westermeyer J, Engdahl B, Johnsen E. 2007. Post-traumatic stress disorder and service utilization in a sample of service members from Iraq and Afghanistan. *Mil Med*. 172:359–363.

Fan F, Zhang Y, Yang Y, et al. 2011. Symptoms of posttraumatic stress disorder, depression, and anxiety among adolescents following the 2008 Wenchuan earthquake in China. *J Trauma Stress.* 24:44–53.

Fear NT, Jones M, Murphy D, et al. 2010. What are the consequences of deployment to Iraq and Afghanistan on the mental health of the UK armed forces? A cohort study. *Lancet.* 375:1783–1797.

Ferrando L, Galea S, Sainz Corton E, et al. 2010. Long-term psychopathology changes among the injured and members of the community after a massive terrorist attack. *Eur Psychiatry.* 26:513–517.

Fiedler N, Ozakinci G, Hallman W, et al. 2006. Military deployment to the Gulf War as a risk factor for psychiatric illness among US troops. *Br J Psychiatry.* 188:453–459.

Friedman MJ, Schnurr PP, McDonagh-Coyle A. 1994. Post-traumatic stress disorder in the military veteran. *Psychiatr Clin North Am.* 17:265–277.

Galea S, Nandi A, Vlahov D. 2005. The epidemiology of post-traumatic stress disorder after disasters. *Epidemiol Rev.* 27:78–91.

Galea S, Vlahov D, Resnick H, et al. 2003. Trends of probable post-traumatic stress disorder in New York City after the September 11 terrorist attacks. *Am J Epidemiol.* 158:514–524.

Grant DM, Beck JG, Marques L, et al. 2008. The structure of distress following trauma: posttraumatic stress disorder, major depressive disorder, and generalized anxiety disorder. *J Abnorm Psychol.* 117:662–672.

Green BL, Korol M, Grace MC, et al. 1991. Children and disaster: age, gender, and parental effects on PTSD symptoms. *J Am Acad Child Adolesc Psychiatry.* 30:945–951.

Grieger TA, Cozza SJ, Ursano RJ, et al. 2006. Posttraumatic stress disorder and depression in battle-injured soldiers. *Am J Psychiatry.* 163:1777–1783.

Harvey AG, Bryant RA. 1998. Relationship of acute stress disorder and posttraumatic stress disorder following motor vehicle accidents. *J Consult Clin Psychol.* 66:507–512.

Hidalgo RB, Davidson JRT. 2000. Posttraumatic stress disorder: epidemiology and health-related considerations. *J Clin Psychiatry.* 61(Suppl 7)5–13.

Hoge CW, Auchterlonie JL, Milliken CS. 2006. Mental health problems, use of mental health services, and attrition from military service after returning from deployment to Iraq or Afghanistan. *JAMA.* 295:1023–1032.

Hoge CW, Castro CA, Messer SC, et al. 2004. Combat duty in Iraq and Afghanistan, mental health problems, and barriers to care. *N Engl J Med.* 351:13–22.

Hoge CW, Terhakopian A, Castro CA, Messer SC, Engel CC. 2007. Association of posttraumatic stress disorder with somatic symptoms, health care visits, and absenteeism among Iraq War Veterans. *Am J Psychiatry.* 164:150–153.

Holmes DT, Tariot PN, Cox C. 1998. Preliminary evidence of psychological distress among reservists in the Persian Gulf War. *J Nerv Ment Dis.* 186:166–173.

Honig RG, Grace MC, Lindy JD, et al. 1993. Portraits of survival. A twenty-year follow-up of the children of Buffalo Creek. *Psychoanal Study Child.* 48:327–355.

Horesch D, Solomon Z, Zerach G, Ein-Dor T. 2010. Delayed-onset PTSD among war veterans: the role of life events throughout the life cycle. *Soc Psychiatry Epidemiol.* 46:863–870.

Kang H, Dalager N, Mahan C, Ishii E. 2005. The role of sexual assault on the risk of PTSD among Gulf War veterans. *Ann Epidemiol.* 15:191–195.

Kang HK, Li B, Mahan CM, et al. 2009. Health of US veterans of the 1991 Gulf War: a follow-up survey in 10 years. *J Occup Environ Med.* 51:401–410.

Kang HK, Natelson BH, Mahan CM, et al. 2003. Post-traumatic stress disorder and chronic fatigue syndrome-like illness among Gulf War veterans: a population-based survey of 30,000 veterans. *Am J Epidemiol.* 157:141–148.

Kennedy JE, Jaffee MS, Leskin GA, et al. 2007. Posttraumatic stress disorder and posttraumatic stress disorder-like symptoms and mild traumatic brain injury. *J Rehabil Res Dev.* 44:895–920.

Kessler DC, Sonnega A, Bromet E, et al. 1995. Posttraumatic stress disorder in the National Comorbidity Survey. *Arch Gen Psychiatry.* 52:1048–1060.

Kessler RC, Berglund P, Demler O, et al. 2005a. Lifetime prevalence and age-at-onset distributions of DSM-IV disorders in the National Comorbidity Survey Replication. *Arch Gen Psychiatry.* 62:593–602.

Kessler RC, Chiu WT, Demler O, et al. 2005b. Prevalence, severity, and comorbidity of 12-month DSM-IV disorders in the National Comorbidity Survey Replication. *Arch Gen Psychiatry.* 62:617–627.

Kilpatrick DG, Ruggiero KJ, Acierno R, et al. 2003. Violence and risk of PTSD, major depression, substance abuse/dependence, and comorbidity: results from the National Survey of Adolescents. *J Consult Clin Psychol.* 71:692–700.

Kimerling R, Gima K, Smith M, et al. 2007. The Veterans Health Administration and military sexual trauma. *Am J Public Health.* 97:2160–2166.

Kimerling R, Street AE, Pavao J, et al. 2010. Military-related sexual trauma among veterans health administration patients returning from Afghanistan and Iraq. *Am J Public Health.* 100:1409–1412.

Kishore V, Theall KP, Robinson W, et al. 2008. Resource loss, coping, alcohol use, and posttraumatic stress symptoms among survivors of Hurricane Katrina: a cross-sectional study. *Am J Disaster Med.* 3:345–357.

Koenen KC, Harley R, Lyons MJ, et al. 2002. A twin registry study of familial and individual risk factors for trauma exposure and posttraumatic stress disorder. *J Nerv Ment Dis.* 190:209–218.

Kohn R, Levav I, Donaire I, et al. 2005. Psychologocial and psychopathological reactions in Honduras following Hurricane Mitch: implications for service planning. *Rev Panam Salud Publica.* 18:287–295.

Kulka RA, Schlenger WE. 1990. The National Vietnam Veterans Readjustment Study: tables of findings and technical appendices. New York: Brunner/Mazel.

Laugharne J, Lillee A, Janca A. 2010. Role of psychological trauma in the cause and treatment of anxiety and depressive disorders. *Curr Opin Psychiatry.* 23:25–29.

Lawson WB. 2009. Anxiety disorders in African Americans and other ethnic minorities. In: Andrews G, Charney DS, Sirovatka PJ, Regier DA, editors. *Stress-induced and fear circuitry disorders. Advancing the research agenda for DSM-V.* Arlington, VA: American Psychiatric Association: 239–244.

LeardMann CA, Smith TC, Smith B, et al. 2009. Baseline self reported functional health and vulnerability to post-traumatic stress disorder after combat deployment: prospective US military cohort study. *BMJ.* 338:b1273. (DOI: 10.1136/bmj.b1273).

Luxton DD, Skopp NA, Maguen S. 2010. Gender differences in depression and PTSD symptoms following combat exposure. *Depress Anxiety.* 27:1027–1033.

MacGregor AJ, Shaffer RA, Dougherty AL, et al. 2009. Psychological correlates of battle and nonbattle injury among Operation Iraqi Freedom veterans. *Mil Med.* 174:224–231.

Marshall RD, Olfson M, Hellman F, et al. 2001. Comorbidity, impairment, and suicidality in subthreshold PTSD. *Am J Psychiatry. 2001*;158:1467–1473.

Martin L, Kagee A. 2011. Lifetime and HIV-related PTSD and persons recently diagnosed with HIV. *AIDS Behav. 2011*;15:125–131.

McFarlane AC. 2010. The long-term costs of traumatic stress: intertwined physical and psychological consequences. *World Psychiatry.* 9:3–10.

Murray J, Ehlers A, Mayou RA. 2002. Dissociation and post-traumatic stress disorder: two prospective studies of road traffic accident survivors. *Br J Psychiatry.* 180:363–368.

Myer L, Smit J, Roux LL, et al. 2008. Common mental disorders among HIV-infected individuals in South Africa: prevalence, predictors, and validation of brief psychiatric rating scales. *AIDS Patient Care STDS.* 22:147–158.

Norris FH, Slone LB. 2007. The epidemiology of trauma and PTSD. In: Friedman MJ, Keane TM, Resick PA, editors. *Handbook of PTSD: Science and practice.* New York: The Guilford Press: 78–98.

North CS, Nixon SJ, Shariat S, et al. 1999. Psychiatric disorders among survivors of the Oklahoma City bombing. *JAMA.* 282:755–762.

North CS, Pferrerbaum B, Narayanan P, et al. 2005. Comparison of post-disaster psychiatric disorders after terrorist bombings in Nairobi and Oklahoma City. *Br J Psychiatry.* 186:487–493.

Pietrzak RH, Goldstein RB, Southwick SM, Grant BF. 2010. Prevalence and Axis I comorbidity of full and partial posttraumatic stress disorder in the United States: results from wave 2 of the National Epidemiologic Survey on Alcohol and Related Conditions. *J Anxiety Disord.* 73:697–707.

Proctor SP, Heeren T, White RF, et al. 1998. Health status of Persian Gulf War veterans: self-reported symptoms, environmental exposures and the effect of stress. *Int J Epidemiol.* 27:1000–1010.

Ramchand R, Karney BR, Osilla KC, et al. 2008. Prevalence of PTSD, depression, and TBI among returning service members. In: Tanielian T, Jaycox LH, editors. *Invisible Wounds: Mental Health and Cognitive Care Needs of America's Returning Veterans.* Santa Monica, CA: RAND Corportion: 35–85.

Resnick HS, Kilpatric DG, Dansky BS, et al. 1993. Prevalence of civilian trauma and posttraumatic stress disorder in a representative national sample of women. *J Consulting Clin Psychology.* 61:984–991.

Roberts AL, Austin SB, Corliss HL, et al. 2010. Pervasive trauma exposure among US sexual orientation minority adults and risk of posttraumatic stress disorder. *Am J Public Health.* 100:2433–2441.

Roberts AL, Gilman SE, Breslau J, et al. 2011a. Race/ethnic differences in exposure to traumatic events, development of post-traumatic stress disorder, and treatment-seeking for post-traumatic stress disorder in the United States. *Psychol Med.* 41:71–83.

Rona RJ, Hooper R, Jones M, et al. 2009. The contribution of prior psychological symptoms and combat exposure to post Iraq deployment mental health in the UK military. *J Trauma Stress.* 22:11–19.

Sadler A, Booth B, Mengeling M, Doebbeling B. 2004. Life span and repeated violence against women during military service: effects on health status and outpatient utilization. *J Women's health.* 13:799–811.

Sadler AG, Booth BM, Cook BL, Doebbeling BN. 2003. Factors associated with women's risk of rape in the military environment. *Am J Ind Med.* 43:262–273.

Sandweiss DA, Slymen DJ, LeardMann CA, et al. 2011. Preinjury psychiatric status, injury severity, and postdeployment posttraumatic stress disorder. *Arch Gen Psychiatry.* 68:496–504.

Schell TL, Marshall GN. 2008. Survey of individuals previously deployed for OIF/OEF. In: Tanielian T, Jaycox LH, editors. *Invisible Wounds: Mental Health and Cognitive Care Needs of America's Returning Veterans.* Santa Monica, CA: RAND Corportion.

Schnyder U, Moergeli H, Klaghofer R, et al. 2001. Incidence and prediction of posttraumatic stress disorder symptoms in severely injured accident victims. *Am J Psychiatry.* 158:594–599.

Schlenger WE, Kulka RA, Fairbank JA, et al. 1992. The prevalence of post-traumatic stress disorder in the Vietnam generation: a multimethod, multisource assessment of psychiatric disorder. *J Traumatic Stress.* 5:333–363.

Schnurr PP, Green BL, editors. 2004. *Trauma and Health: Physical Consequences of Exposure to Extreme Stress.* Washington, DC: American Psychological Association.

Seal KH, Bertenthal D, Miner CR, et al. 2007. Bringing the war back home: mental health disorders among 103,788 U.S. veterans returning from Iraq and

Afghanistan seen at Department of Veterans Affairs facilities. *Arch Intern Med.* 167:476–482.

Shen YC, Arkes J, Pilgrim J. 2009. The effects of deployment intensity on post-traumatic stress disorder: 2002-2006. *Mil Med.* 174:217–223.

Steele L. 2000. Prevalence and patterns of Gulf War illness in Kansas veterans: association of symptoms with characteristics of person, place, and time of military service. *Am J Epidemiol.* 152:992–1002.

Smith TC, Ryan MAK, Wingard DL, et al. 2008. New onset and persistent symptoms of post-traumatic stress disorder self reported after deployment and combat exposures: prospective population based US military cohort study. *BMJ.* 336:366–371.

Smith TC, Wingard DL, Ryan MAK, et al. 2009. PTSD prevalence, associated exposures, and functional health outcomes in a large, population-based military cohort. *Public Health Rep.* 124:90–102.

Stein MB, Walker JR, Hazen AL, Forde DR. 1997. Full and partial posttraumatic stress disorder: findings from a community survey. *Am J Psychiatry.* 154:1114–1119.

Suris A, Lind L, Kashner M, et al. 2008. Sexual assault in women veterans: an examination of PTSD risk, health care utilization, and cost of care. *Psychosomatic Med.* 66:749–756.

Suris A, Lind L. Military sexual trauma. A review of prevalence and associated health consequences in veterans. 2008. *Trauma Violence Abuse.* 9:250–269.

Terhakopian A, Sinaii N, Engel CC, Schnurr PP, Hoge CW. 2008. Estimating population prevalence of posttraumatic stress disorder: an example using the PTSD checklist. *J Traumatic Stress.* 21:290–300.

Toomey R, Kang HK, Karlinsky J, et al. 2007. Mental health of US Gulf War veterans 10 years after the war. *Br J Psychiatry.* 190:385–393.

Vasterling JJ, Proctor SP, Friedman MJ, et al. 2010. PTSD symptom increases in Iraq-deployed soldiers: comparison with nondeployed soldiers and associations with baseline symptoms, deployment experiences, and postdeployment stress. *J Trauma Stress.* 23:41–51.

Vasterling JJ, Schumm J, Proctor SP, et al. 2008. Posttraumatic stress disorder and health functioning in a non-treatment-seeking sample of Iraq war veterans: a prospective analysis. *J Rehabil Res Dev.* 45:347–358.

Verger P, Dab W, Lamping DL, et al. 2004. The psychological impact of terrorism: an epidemiologic study of posttraumatic stress disorder and associated factors in victims of the 1995–1996 bombings in France. *Am J Psychiatry.* 161:1384–1389.

Vogt D, Smith B, Elwy R, et al. 2011. Predeployment, deployment, and postdeployment risk factors for posttraumatic stress symptomatology in female and male OEF/OIF veterans. *J Abnorm Psychol.* 120:919–931.

Vogt D, Vaughn R, Glickman ME, et al. 2011. Gender differences in combat-related stressors and their association with postdeployment mental health in a nationally representative sample of U.S. OEF/OIF veterans. *J Abnorm Psychol.* 120:797–806.

Weathers FW, Litz BT, Herman DS, et al. 1993. The PTSD Checklist (PCL): reliability, validity, and diagnostic utility. Presented at the annual convention of the International Society for Traumatic Stress Studies, San Antonio, Texas, October 1993.

Wolfe J, Erickson DJ, Sharkansky EJ, et al. 1999. Course and predictors of posttraumatic stress disorder among Gulf War veterans: a prospective analysis. *J Consult Clin Psychol.* 67:520–528.

Yang P, Yen CF, Tang TC, et al. 2010. Posttraumatic stress disorder in adolescents after Typhoon Morakot-associated mudslides. *J Anxiety Disord.* 25:362–368.

3

Post-Traumatic Stress Disorder and Other Psychiatric Conditions

Steven S. Coughlin, Ph.D.

This chapter summarizes the literature on the co-occurrence of Post-Traumatic Stress Disorder (PTSD) and other psychiatric conditions. Population surveys and clinical studies have shown that comorbid conditions are common among persons with PTSD. In the National Comorbidity Survey (Kessler et al. 1995), 88% of men and 79% of women with PTSD met criteria for at least one other psychiatric diagnosis. Similar comorbidity rates have been observed in other population surveys (Breslau et al. 1992; Creamer et al. 2001). In addition to PTSD, traumatic events increase vulnerability to several psychiatric disorders including generalized anxiety disorder, acute anxiety disorder, major depressive disorder as well as other mood disorders, eating disorders, and borderline personality disorder. In addition, there are some shared risk factors across various anxiety and mood disorders (Laugharne et al. 2010). Persons who have PTSD-type symptoms may receive a different diagnosis (for example, panic disorder or major depressive disorder) because they have either not experienced a severe enough stressor or they have insufficient symptoms to make the full PTSD diagnosis (Laugharne et al. 2010). As a result of these and other complexities, there has been ongoing discussion in the psychiatric and psychological literature about how best to define PTSD and other anxiety and mood disorders that may result from trauma or shared vulnerabilities (Friedman et al. 2010; Rosen et al. 2008). Comorbidity with other anxiety disorders and mood disorders are discussed below along with other Axis I and Axis II psychiatric comorbidities. Substance abuse and dependence are discussed separately in Chapter 5. The co-occurrence of PTSD and traumatic brain injury, which has also been associated with anxiety and depression, is discussed in Chapter 8.

ANXIETY DISORDERS

Anxiety disorders are common in the general population and in patient samples. Epidemiologic and clinical studies have shown that PTSD is associated with increased rates of anxiety disorders including social phobia, agoraphobia, specific phobia, obsessive-compulsive disorder, and somatization disorder. As noted in the Diagnostic and Statistical Manual of Mental Disorders (DSM-IV), these Axis I disorders can precede, follow, or emerge at the same time as the onset of PTSD. There is often symptom overlap between PTSD and other anxiety disorders.

Generalized Anxiety Disorder

Generalized anxiety disorder is characterized by persistent and excessive anxiety and worry over a period of at least 6 months (DSM-IV). Symptoms of this disorder include restlessness, being easily fatigued, difficulty concentrating, irritability, muscle tension, and sleep disturbance (DSM-IV). According to DSM-IV criteria, generalized anxiety disorder is not diagnosed if the anxiety occurs exclusively during the course of PTSD. Kessler and Wittchen (2002) noted that the high comorbidity of generalized anxiety disorder with other anxiety and mood disorders in clinical samples may be due to the higher levels of distress experienced by patients with psychiatric comorbidity. Persons experiencing greater distress may be more likely to seek care (Kessler and Wittchen 2002). Studies of persons traumatized by motor vehicle accidents, natural disasters such as hurricanes and earthquakes, armed conflict, and other severe stressors have shown that PTSD, generalized anxiety disorder, and major depressive disorder can occur among persons exposed to traumatic events and that it is possible to distinguish between these psychiatric conditions (Grant et al. 2008; Acierno et al. 2007). The co-occurrence of PTSD and major depressive disorder is discussed later in this chapter.

Acute Stress Disorder

Acute stress disorder occurs within four weeks of a traumatic event and is characterized by symptoms similar to those seen in PTSD, but with acute stress disorder more emphasis is placed on dissociative reactions to the trauma (DSM-IV). Although the temporal definitions of acute stress disorder and PTSD preclude them from overlapping, persons with acute stress disorder are at increased risk for developing PTSD at a later point in time. Bryant (2010) recently reviewed 22 studies (19 with adults and three with children) that had assessed acute stress disorder within four weeks of trauma exposure and later assessed PTSD. The rates of acute stress disorder ranged from 7–59% across studies, with a mean of 17%. The majority of trauma survivors who eventually developed PTSD did not meet the full criteria for acute stress disorder. In the 19 studies of adults, at least half of those trauma survivors with acute stress disorder subsequently met criteria for PTSD (Bryant 2010). Results from the three studies of children suggest that acute stress disorder is a poor predictor of PTSD in injured children (Bryant 2010). Fullerton et al. (2004) studied acute stress disorder, PTSD, and depression in disaster or rescue workers (n = 207) who had been exposed to an airline disaster. A comparison group of 421 unexposed workers was included. The exposed and unexposed disaster workers were assessed at 2, 7, and 13 months after the crash in which many passengers were killed or seriously wounded. Acute stress disorder during the first week after the disaster was assessed at two months. Exposed disaster workers had higher rates of acute stress disorder, PTSD at 13 months, depression at 7 months, and depression at 13 months than comparison workers. Exposed disaster workers with acute stress disorder were 7.3 times more likely to develop PTSD (95% confidence interval = 2.5–21.3) during the course of the study (Fullerton et al. 2004).

Phobia

Phobias include specific phobia (e.g., fear of animals, flying, or receiving an injection), social phobia (e.g., fear of social or performance situations), and agoraphobia, or anxiety about places or situations from which escape might be difficult or embarrassing (e.g., being in an elevator or traveling in a bus or automobile), or avoidance of such places (DSM-IV). Persons with agoraphobia may avoid a variety of situations out of fear of having panic-like symptoms and not having help available or being embarrassed. In the DSM-IV, criterion C for agoraphobia requires that the anxiety or phobic avoidance not be better accounted for by another mental disorder including social phobia, specific phobia, or PTSD (e.g., the avoidance of stimuli associated with a severe stressor or trauma). Similarly, DSM-IV criterion G for specific phobia requires that the anxiety or phobic avoidance associated with the specific object or situation not be better accounted for by another mental disorder including social phobia or PTSD. However, specific phobias are frequently comorbid with other anxiety and mood disorders (DSM-IV). The cooccurrence of PTSD and phobia has been examined in veterans (Orsillo et al. 1996; Crowson et al. 1998; Hofmann et al. 2003), in motor vehicle accident survivors (Mayou et al. 2001), and in victims of terrorist attacks (Handley et al. 2009). Orsillo et al. (1996) assessed 41 Vietnam combat veterans and found that 32% had comorbid PTSD and social phobia. Symptoms of social phobia or social anxiety experienced by combat veterans with PTSD may be mediated by major depression (Hofmann et al. 2003). Handley et al. (2009) analyzed data from a screening and treatment program that was set up to provide rapid assessment and treatment for persons directly affected by the July 7, 2005, terrorist bombings in London. About 45% of the 596 respondents to the screening program reported phobic fear of public transport. The screening program identified 255 bombing survivors who needed treatment for a psychological disorder. Of these, 20 (8%) suffered from clinically significant travel phobia. Many of these individuals also reported PTSD symptoms, raising the possibility that travel phobia in these individuals may represent subthreshold PTSD or a milder version of PTSD (Handley et al. 2009).

Panic Disorder

Panic attacks consist of the sudden onset of intense fear and apprehension, in the absence of real danger, and are often associated with feelings of impending death and an urge to escape (DSM-IV). Cognitive and somatic symptoms such as shortness of breath, heart palpitations, and feeling lightheaded or faint commonly occur during panic attacks. Recurrent unexpected panic attacks are required for a diagnosis of panic disorder. Persons with PTSD may suffer from panic attacks when exposed to stimuli that remind them of their trauma (Brady et al. 2000). In an analysis of data from the National Comorbidity Survey Replication, Cougle et al. (2010) found that 203 respondents met DSM-IV criteria for PTSD in the past year. About 35% of the 203 respondents with PTSD had panic attacks within the past year. In the Epidemiologic Catchment Area survey conducted in St. Louis in 1981, in which members of randomly sampled households were interviewed, women with PTSD had a fourfold increased risk of having panic disorder as compared with women who did not have PTSD (Helzer et al. 1987). No increased risk of panic disorder was observed among men with PTSD, however (Helzer et al. 1987). Engdahl et al. (1998) observed a strong association between PTSD and panic disorder in a study of 140 veterans who had been prisoners of war. The odds ratio for current PTSD was about 13.7 (Engdahl et al. 1998).

Obsessive-Compulsive Disorder

Obsessive-compulsive disorder is characterized either by recurrent and persistent thoughts, impulses, or images (i.e., obsessions) that are experienced as intrusive and inappropriate, or compulsions such as excessive hand washing, cleaning, checking, or counting (DSM-IV). The obsessions or compulsions cause pronounced distress and interfere with the person's occupational functioning, social activities, or relationships. In contrast to PTSD-related flashbacks, the recurrent intrusive thoughts that may occur in obsessive-compulsive disorder are not related to an experienced traumatic event (DSM-IV). Nevertheless, symptom overlap may artificially increase the co-occurrence of PTSD and obsessive-compulsive disorder (Huppert et al. 2005). The co-occurrence of PTSD and obsessive-compulsive disorder has been examined in clinical samples and in population surveys (Helzer et al. 1987; Breslau et al. 1991; Davidson et al. 1991; Huppert et al. 2005; Gershuny et al. 2008). Huppert et al. (2005) examined the relationship between these two disorders in 128 patients diagnosed with obsessive-compulsive disorder and 109 patients diagnosed with PTSD. Overall symptoms of obsessive-compulsive disorder and PTSD were related in the patient groups. However, after controlling for overlapping symptoms and depression, the relationship was no longer significant (Huppert et al. 2005). In the Epidemiologic Catchment Area survey conducted in St. Louis, persons with PTSD had a 10-fold increased risk of having obsessive-compulsive disorder as compared with persons without PTSD (Helzer et al. 1987).

MOOD DISORDERS

This section considers the co-occurrence of PTSD and major depressive disorder, which has also been referred to as clinical depression. The co-occurrence of PTSD and bipolar disorders, which are also important comorbid conditions, is discussed separately below.

Major Depressive Disorder

Major depressive disorder is characterized by one or more major depressive episodes with five or more symptoms of depression such as depressed mood, loss of interest or pleasure in all or most daily activities, significant weight loss or gain, sleeping disturbances, fatigue or loss of energy, feelings of worthlessness or excessive or inappropriate guilt, diminished ability to think or concentrate, or recurrent thoughts of death or suicidal ideation (DSM-IV). The key feature of major depressive disorder is a period of at least 2 weeks during which there is either depressed mood or a loss of interest or pleasure in all or nearly all activities. For a diagnosis of major depressive disorder to be made, the symptoms must cause significant distress or impairment in social, occupational, or other areas of functioning, and not be due to a general medical condition or medication (DSM-IV). In addition, there must never have been a manic or hypomanic episode. According to the DSM-IV, major depressive disorder may be mild, moderate, or severe; severe depressive disorder may occur with or without psychosis. The International Classification of Diseases (ICD-10) includes separate codes to indicate whether the current episode of recurrent depressive disorder is mild, moderate, severe without psychotic symptoms, or severe with psychotic symptoms.

Major depressive disorder occurs frequently after traumatic exposures, both by itself or concurrently with PTSD (O'Donnell et al. 2004). About 30–50% of persons diagnosed with PTSD have symptoms of depression (Kessler et al. 1995; Boudreaux et al. 1998; Campbell et al. 2007). The prevalence of dysthymia has also been reported to be increased among persons with PTSD (Helzer et al. 1987; Breslau et al. 1991; Kessler et al. 1995). The co-occurrence of PTSD and major depressive disorder has been observed in population surveys (Helzer et al. 1987; Davidson et al. 1991; Kessler et al. 1995) and samples of clinic patients (Stein et al. 2000; Nixon et al. 2004; Hegel et al. 2005; Mittal et al. 2006; Campbell et al. 2007; Liebschutz et al. 2007; Lowe et al.

2010). In addition to clinic patients and members of the general population, studies documenting PTSD-major depression comorbidity have focused on veterans (Zatzick et al. 1997; Mittal et al. 2006; Campbell et al. 2007; Chan et al. 2009; Ginzburg et al. 2010; Gros et al. 2010; Ikin et al. 2010), women who were the victim of intimate partner violence (Boudreaux et al. 1998; Stein and Kennedy 2001; Nixon et al. 2004; Taft et al. 2009), persons suffering injuries from motor vehicle accidents or other severe trauma (O'Donnell et al. 2004), and disaster or rescue workers (Fullerton et al. 2004). People with comorbid PTSD and major depressive disorder have been reported to have impaired health-related quality of life as compared with those with major depressive disorder alone (Mittal et al. 2006; Ikin et al. 2010). The cooccurrence of major depressive disorder and anxiety disorders has been associated with poorer prognosis, greater duration and severity of depressive illness, poorer treatment response, and higher risk of suicide (Brown et al. 1996; Oquendo et al. 2005; Mittal et al. 2006; Campbell et al. 2007; Chan et al. 2009). Comorbid major depression may be an important mediator of the reported association between PTSD and somatization disorder (Davidson et al. 1991; Lowe et al. 2010). The co-occurrence of PTSD and major depression has also been well documented in persons living with HIV/AIDS, cancer, and other potentially life-threatening illnesses (Smith et al. 1999; Kangas et al. 2005; Olley et al. 2005; Myer et al. 2008; Whetten et al. 2008).

Hegel et al. (2005) examined the effect of comorbid PTSD and panic disorder on depression treatment outcomes among older primary care patients (n = 1,801) who suffered from depression. At baseline, the co-occurrence of PTSD, panic disorder, and depression was associated with impaired quality of life and greater functional impairment as compared with depression alone (Hegel et al. 2005). Campbell et al. (2007) examined comorbidity from PTSD and depression in a random sample of 677 patients treated for depression at Veterans Health Administration primary care practices. At baseline, 36% of the depressed patients screened positive for PTSD. Patients with comorbid PTSD and depression reported more severe depression, lower social support, and more frequent outpatient health care visits, and were more likely to report suicidal ideation than those with depression alone (Campbell et al. 2007). The authors noted that some patients with PTSD and major depressive disorder might have been misidentified and that it was unclear which illness was primary (Campbell et al. 2007). Relatively few longitudinal studies of PTSD and depression have been reported (Breslau and Davis 1992; O'Donnell et al. 2004; Ginzburg et al. 2010; Neria et al. 2010). Neria et al. (2010) examined the mental health effects of the Israel-Gaza War (2008–2009) among young adult civilians in Southern Israel (n = 200). Information about PTSD, major depressive disorder, and generalized anxiety disorder was collected during the war, and again at two and four months after the ceasefire. A sharp decline in levels of PTSD, major depressive disorder, and generalized anxiety disorder was observed over time (Neria et al. 2010). Ginzburg et al. (2010) examined 664 Israeli veterans of the 1982 Lebanon War following up 1, 2, and 20 years after their wartime experiences. At each assessment, rates of comorbid PTSD-anxiety-depression (26.7–30.1%) were higher than rates of PTSD alone (9.3–11.1%). PTSD predicted depression and comorbid disorders but not vice versa (Ginzburg et al. 2010).

In the general population of the United States and many other countries, the prevalence of major depressive disorder is higher among women than men. Studies have suggested that gender may mediate the associations between traumatic exposures (e.g., those experienced during combat or natural disasters such as earthquakes) and both depression and PTSD (Luxton et al. 2010; Dell'osso et al. 2011; Fan et al. 2011). For example, Luxton et al. (2010) reported that combat exposures may be a stronger predictor of post-deployment depression and PTSD for women than men.

Mood disorders and PTSD have some symptoms in common including symptoms related to emotional numbing and dysphoria (Gros et al. 2010). Shared symptomatology may partly account for the co-occurrence of PTSD and major depressive disorder (Gros et al. 2010). When PTSD and depression occur together, they may reflect a shared vulnerability (O'Donnell et al. 2004). Persons with PTSD are more likely to develop major depressive disorder (Breslau et al. 1997; Fullerton et al. 2004; Ginzburg et al. 2010; Wells et al. 2010). However, the reverse may also be true. Those people with preexisting major depressive disorder may be more susceptible to developing PTSD following a traumatic event (Breslau et al. 1991; Oquendo et al. 2005).

Neurobiological and neuroimaging studies have identified differences between PTSD and major depressive disorder, and between comorbid PTSD-major depression and PTSD alone (Yehuda et al. 1996; Lanius et al. 2007; Kandwerger 2009; Gill et al. 2010). Gill et al. (2010) reported that PTSD patients who had comorbid major depressive disorder (n = 9) had higher interleukin-6 levels than PTSD patients who did not have major depressive disorder (n = 9) and healthy control subjects (n = 14). The patients with PTSD alone had greater sensitivity to intravenous hydrocortisone than those with comorbid PTSD-major depressive disorder (Gill et al. 2010). Although both PTSD and major depression may occur following traumatic events, the hypothalamic-pituitary-adrenal function abnormalities seen in PTSD and major depressive disorder have been reported to be distinct (Handwerger 2009).

Bipolar Disorders

Epidemiologic studies have found that bipolar disorders cooccur with PTSD and other anxiety disorders at rates that are higher than those in the general population (Kessler et al. 1997; Freeman et al. 2002). In the National Comorbidity Survey Replication, about 31% of the participants who met criteria for lifetime bipolar I disorder had PTSD (Merikangas et al. 2007). About 34% of those who met criteria for lifetime bipolar II disorder had PTSD. Neria et al. (2008) examined relationships between exposure to trauma, bipolar disorder and PTSD in a sample of 977 adult primary care patients from a general medicine practice in New York City. Adjustment was made in the analysis for age group, income level, positive screen for current alcohol or drug use disorder, and screen for current major depressive episode. Patients who screened positive for bipolar disorder were 2.6 times (95% confidence interval 1.6–4.2) more likely to report physical or sexual assault than those who screened negative for bipolar disorder (Neria et al. 2008). In addition, those who screened positive for bipolar disorder were 2.9 times (95% confidence interval 1.6–5.1) more likely to screen positive for current PTSD (Neria et al. 2008). Bipolar illness might be a consequence of early traumatic events such as physical or sexual assault during childhood (Neria et al. 2008). After its onset, bipolar illness may also lead to additional traumatic events (Otto et al. 2004).

The coexistence of PTSD and other Axis I disorders with bipolar disorder may be associated with a more severe course, poorer treatment compliance, and worse outcomes (Krishnan 2005; Quarantini et al. 2010). Once developed, PTSD is likely to have an adverse effect on the course of bipolar disorder including elevated rates of suicide attempts and lower quality of life (Otto et al. 2004). Quarantini et al. (2010) studied 405 patients with bipolar disorder seen at two teaching hospitals in Brazil. Those who had comorbid PTSD reported worse quality of life, more rapid cycling, and greater numbers of suicide attempts than bipolar disorder patients without PTSD (Quarantini et al. 2010).

In addition to traumatic life events and adverse experiences, neurobiological and genetic factors may account for the co-occurrence of bipolar disorder and PTSD. The neurobiological mechanisms that explain comorbidity between bipolar disorder and PTSD may involve a complex interplay among neurotransmitter systems in the brain, such as those involving norepinephrine, dopamine, gamma-aminobutyric acid, and serotonin (Freeman et al. 2002).

EATING DISORDERS

Eating disorders such as anorexia nervosa (with reluctance to maintain a minimally normal body weight and intense fear of gaining weight) and bulimia nervosa (recurrent episodes of binge eating and inappropriate compensatory behavior to prevent weight gain) have been associated with a variety of traumatic experiences including childhood sexual abuse and other forms of physical abuse and neglect (Brewerton 2007). The spectrum of traumatic experiences associated with eating disorders includes sexual assault during adulthood, sexual harassment, physical assault, emotional abuse, and bullying (Brewerton 2007). A history of trauma is more common in bulimic eating disorders than in nonbulimic eating disorders. Trauma is associated with greater comorbidity from PTSD and other Axis I and Axis II disorders in eating disorder patients (Brewerton 2007). Although eating disorders are more common among women than men, eating disorders associated with traumatic experiences also occur among men, and among children and adolescents.

Clinical studies of women seeking treatment for eating disorders have shown that PTSD is a common comorbid condition (Gleaves et al. 1998; Tagay et al. 2010). Epidemiologic studies also show that PTSD and eating disorders frequently co-occur. In the National Women's Study (Dansky et al. 1997), the lifetime prevalence rate of PTSD was 37% among participants with bulimia nervosa as compared with 12% among those without an eating disorder. In that study from the 1990s, the current prevalence rate of PTSD was 21% in participants with bulimia nervosa as compared with 4% among those without an eating disorder (Dansky et al. 1997). Dobie et al. (2004) surveyed women (n = 1,935) who received care at the Department of Veterans Affairs Puget Sound

Health Care System between October 1996 and January 1998. The survey included questions about medical history and health habits. The PTSD Checklist-Civilian Version (PCL-C) was included. Of the 1,259 eligible women who completed the survey, 266 (21%) screened positive for current PTSD (PCL-C score $\geq$ 50). About 25% (66 of 266) of women with PTSD screened positive for an eating disorder compared with 6% (60 of 940) of women without PTSD (age-adjusted odds ratio = 5.0, 95% confidence interval 3.4–7.4). About 47% (124 of 263) of women with PTSD screened positive for panic disorder compared with 4% (37 of 926) of women without PTSD (age-adjusted odds ratio = 21.4, 95% confidence interval 14.1–32.4).

Clinical studies have shown that eating disorder patients who have experienced traumatic events are more likely to drop out of treatment and have higher relapse rates than eating disorder patients without a trauma history (Mahon et al. 2001; Rodriguez et al. 2005). There is currently a paucity of studies of treatment outcomes among patients with comorbid PTSD and eating disorders, however.

BORDERLINE PERSONALITY DISORDER

In contrast to PTSD and other Axis I disorders, borderline personality disorder is an Axis II disorder in the DSM-IV. However, both PTSD and borderline personality disorder have important relationships with traumatic experiences (Pagura et al. 2010). Persons with borderline personality disorder often have a history of trauma including childhood physical and sexual abuse (Herman et al. 1989; Zanarini et al. 1989; Ogata et al. 1990). However, exposure to a traumatic event is not required for a diagnosis of borderline personality disorder to be made. Clinical studies of treatment-seeking individuals and epidemiologic studies have shown that borderline personality disorder is associated with substantial medical comorbidity, functional impairment, impaired quality of life, and increased healthcare utilization (Black et al. 2006; Pagura et al. 2010). Recurrent suicidal threats and self-harm behaviors (for example, cutting and burning) are frequently seen among borderline personality disorder patients and such behaviors are among the core diagnostic criteria for the disorder. Other criteria for borderline personality disorder relate to inappropriate anger or difficulty controlling anger, impulsivity, affective instability, frantic efforts to avoid real or imagined abandonment, unstable relationships, chronic feelings of emptiness, identity disturbance with unstable self-image, and transient paranoid ideation, delusions, or dissociative symptoms. Only five of the nine criteria are required for a diagnosis of borderline personality disorder.

Clinical studies and population surveys have shown that 25–58% of persons with borderline personality disorder have PTSD (Famularo et al. 1991; Hudziak et al. 1996; Zanarini et al. 1998; Zimmerman and Mattia 1999; Yen et al. 2002; Zlotnick et al. 2002; Golier et al. 2003; Harned et al. 2008; Pagura et al. 2010). Although comorbidity estimates vary across settings, studies also show that a sizeable percentage of persons who seek clinical treatment for PTSD have borderline personality disorder (Zlotnick et al. 2002; Southwick et al. 1993). Studies also document that some veterans with combat-related PTSD have borderline personality disorder or features of the disorder (Southwick et al. 1993; Axelrod et al. 2005; Black et al. 2006).

Connor et al. (2002) examined the impact of borderline personality disorder on PTSD in a community survey. A total of 150 adult respondents had a lifetime history of PTSD. On average, those with both PTSD and borderline personality disorder (n = 15) had greater functional impairment and poorer health status, and were more likely to utilize mental health services. Pagura et al. (2010) examined comorbid borderline personality disorder and PTSD in the general U.S. population using data from the National Epidemiologic Survey on Alcohol and Related Conditions Wave II. The lifetime prevalence of PTSD and borderline personality disorder were 6.6% (95% confidence interval 6.3–7.0%) and 5.9% (95% confidence interval 5.5–6.3%), respectively. About 30.2% of persons with borderline personality disorder were also diagnosed with PTSD (Pagura et al. 2010). About 24.2% of persons with PTSD were also diagnosed with borderline personality disorder (Pagura et al. 2010). In the large national survey, persons with comorbid PTSD and borderline personality disorder (n = 643, population prevalence = 1.6%, 95% confidence interval 1.4–1.8%) had a poorer quality of life, more comorbidity with other Axis I conditions, and an increased odds of a lifetime suicide attempt than those with PTSD or borderline personality disorder alone (Pagura et al. 2010). People with comorbid PTSD and borderline personality disorder also reported the highest number of PTSD symptoms, on average, than those with PTSD alone or borderline personality disorder alone (Pagura et al. 2010).

Trauma during childhood may affect personality development in a way that increases vulnerability for developing PTSD later in life (Gunderson and Sabo 1993). Higher rates of PTSD in persons with borderline personality disorder may reflect a diminished ability to adapt to or recover from traumatic events (Golier et al. 2003). Studies have shown that adverse experiences during childhood increase risk for subsequent PTSD (Bremner et al. 1993; Widom 1999; Cabrera et al. 2007). Borderline personality disorder features may also develop in response to PTSD symptoms. For example, chronic insomnia and nightmares can lead to irritability, intense anger, and mood changes (Axelrod et al. 2005).

There have been some critiques of the borderline personality disorder diagnosis including concerns that the disorder may be overdiagnosed among female patients or that the word "borderline" is inaccurate or pejorative (Vaillant 1992). Alternative terminology and definitions for the disorder have been proposed. For example, suggestions for reformulating complex PTSD and borderline personality disorder were outlined by Classen et al. (2006). Although some authors have argued that borderline personality disorder should be subsumed into PTSD, evidence from clinical studies suggests that the two conditions are distinct but that they may be comorbid in some individuals. For example, Zanarini et al. (1998) found that about 56% of patients with borderline personality disorder (212 of 379) had PTSD, which is inconsistent with the view that borderline personality disorder should be conceptualized as a chronic form of PTSD. Some studies suggest that patients who have both PTSD and borderline personality disorder may have a particularly severe and complex clinical presentation, although results have been somewhat inconsistent (Heffernan and Cloitre 2000; Zlotnick et al. 2002; Zlotnick et al. 2003; Harned et al. 2010). Harned et al. (2010) studied 94 female patients with borderline personality disorder who had recently attempted suicide or exhibited self-injurious behavior. One group of patients (n = 53) had a comorbid diagnosis of PTSD and the other group (n = 41) did not. Several differences were found between the two groups. Those with both PTSD and borderline personality disorder were more likely to utilize intentional self-injury as a means to influence others. Patients with both PTSD and borderline personality disorder were almost two times as likely to report unwanted sexual experiences than those with only borderline personality disorder (Harned et al. 2010). Those with both PTSD and borderline personality disorder had greater impairment than those with borderline personality disorder alone. The authors noted that a vacillation between intense emotional re-experiencing (e.g., flashbacks and distressing memories of the trauma) and emotional numbing seen in PTSD may exacerbate the emotion dysregulation that is a core feature of borderline personality disorder (Harned et al. 2010).

Studies have suggested that the neurobiological pathways that account for comorbid PTSD and borderline personality disorder may relate to the hypothalamic-pituitary-adrenal axis (Southwick et al. 2003; Lange et al. 2005; Jogems-Kosterman et al. 2007; Wingenfeld et al. 2007a, 2007b).

ANTISOCIAL PERSONALITY DISORDER

The prevalence of antisocial personality disorder is about 3–5% in the general U.S. population (Robins et al. 1991; Goodwin and Hamilton 2003; Compton et al. 2005). Diagnostic criteria for antisocial personality disorder include a pervasive disregard for and violation of the rights of others as indicated by failure to conform to social norms (lawful behaviors), deceitfulness, impulsivity, irritability and aggressiveness, reckless disregard for the safety of self or others, consistent irresponsibility, and lack of remorse (DSM-IV). Antisocial personality disorder is more common among men than women (Zlotnick et al. 2001; Goldstein et al. 2010). Epidemiologic studies have shown that 8–21% of persons with PTSD have antisocial personality disorder (Jordan et al. 1991; Barrett et al. 1996; Goodwin and Hamilton 2003). Similar percentages have been reported in clinical studies of patients seeking treatment for PTSD in non-substance use disorder treatment settings (Bollinger et al. 2000; Zlotnick et al. 2001; Dunn et al. 2004).

SCHIZOPHRENIA AND PSYCHOSIS

Several studies have examined PTSD among persons with schizophrenia or other psychotic disorders (Shaw et al. 1997; Sautter et al. 1999; Resnick et al. 2003; Mueser et al. 2004; Calhoun et al. 2006). Calhoun et al. (2006) examined the impact of comorbid PTSD on health-related quality of life and health care utilization in 165 male veterans with primary schizophrenia who had been admitted to a Veterans Affairs inpatient psychiatric unit. Comorbid PTSD was associated with decreased quality of life and increased health care utilization including psychiatric hospitalizations and outpatient visits for physical health complaints (Calhoun et al. 2006). About 41% (67 of 165) of the patients screened positive for PTSD based upon a score of 50 or higher on the Posttraumatic Stress Disorder Checklist (PCL-17). Although the generalizability of these findings is uncertain, these results do suggest that PTSD is an important comorbid disorder among veterans who have schizophrenia (Calhoun et al. 2006).

The co-occurrence of PTSD and schizophrenia and other forms of severe mental illness has also been examined in non-veteran samples. Mueser et al. (2004) examined the prevalence of PTSD in persons with severe mental illness who were receiving services in one of five inpatient and outpatient treatment settings. The patients were selected using a combination of convenience sampling and probability sampling. All of the patients had a diagnosis of schizophrenia, other psychotic disorder, or major mood disorder. In the subset of patients with schizophrenia (n = 363), the current prevalence of PTSD was about 29% (Mueser et al. 2004). Taken overall, findings to date indicate that PTSD is one of the most common comorbid conditions in people with severe mental illness (Mueser et al. 2004; Calhoun et al. 2006). As noted by Brady et al. (2000), persons with chronic mental illness are likely to be a particularly vulnerable population at high risk for traumatic events and subsequent PTSD due to unstable living conditions, poor interpersonal skills, and impaired cognitive status. Studies have shown that traumatic life events such as sexual and physical abuse and assault are common among persons with schizophrenia and other forms of severe mental illness (Mueser et al. 2002; Shaw et al. 1997).

Mueser et al. (2002) posited that PTSD may influence schizophrenia and other forms of severe mental illness through both direct and indirect effects. Factors commonly associated with PTSD (for example, substance abuse and difficulty with interpersonal relationships) may adversely affect the course of schizophrenia. In addition, PTSD may directly influence schizophrenia through PTSD symptoms such as avoidance and reexperiencing phenomena (Mueser et al. 2002). Intrusive memories of traumatic events may aggravate the underlying psychotic illness (Shaw et al. 1997).

In some patients, PTSD may represent a response to the traumatic experience of psychotic illness or hospitalization, that is, post-psychosis PTSD. Shaw et al. (1997) examined PTSD symptoms in 45 patients with schizophrenia or other psychotic illness who were between the ages of 16 and 65 years. All of the patients were recovering from hospitalization for a psychotic episode. They were recruited from a general hospital psychiatric unit and the acute admission ward of a large psychiatric hospital. Psychotic symptoms such as persecutory delusions and visual hallucinations and certain treatment experiences (for example, involuntary detention, seclusion, and closed ward care) were perceived as highly distressing. Overall, 22 (45%) of the subjects met study criteria for post-psychosis PTSD (Shaw et al. 1997).

A further possibility is that PTSD with psychotic features may be a particularly severe subtype of PTSD (David et al. 1999; Hamner et al. 1999; Sautter et al. 1999; Braakman et al. 2009). In a recent review of the evidence from clinical studies about the validity of 'PTSD with secondary psychotic features,' Braakman et al. (2009) noted that studies have not found a relationship between psychotic features in PTSD and alcohol or drug dependence. Clinical studies do show that PTSD may co-occur with auditory hallucinations or delusional thought processes (Sautter et al. 1999; Braakman et al. 2009). There is some evidence from neurobiological research suggesting that PTSD with secondary psychotic features may be a distinct diagnostic entity (Sautter et al. 2003; Braakman et al. 2008). For example, cerebrospinal fluid concentrations of corticotrophin-releasing factor have been reported to be higher in patients with PTSD with secondary psychotic symptoms than in PTSD patients without psychotic symptoms and healthy controls ($p < 0.01$) (Sautter et al. 2003).

SUMMARY AND CONCLUSIONS

The published studies reviewed in this chapter underscore the important psychiatric comorbidity that can be seen among persons exposed to traumatic events such as combat exposures, sexual assault, physical abuse, terrorist attacks, natural disasters, or motor vehicle accidents resulting in severe trauma. The co-occurrence of PTSD and other psychiatric disorders (including alcohol and substance dependence discussed in the chapter that follows) is partly due to shared risk factors and the fact that traumatic events can lead to more than one condition in the same individual (for example, comorbid PTSD and major depressive disorder). Symptom overlap also contributes to comorbidity, such as when persons with PTSD suffer from panic attacks when exposed to stimuli that remind them of their traumatic experiences (Brady et al. 2000). Other explanations for comorbidity include the observations that persons with PTSD are more likely to develop major depressive disorder and, conversely, persons with preexisting major depressive disorder and certain other psychiatric disorders may have greater vulnerability to developing PTSD following a traumatic event (Breslau et al. 1997; Oquendo et al. 2005; Ginzburg et al. 2010; Wells et al. 2010). Persons with bipolar disorder or schizophrenia may experience additional traumatic events and be at high risk of developing PTSD (Mueser et al. 2004; Otto et al. 2004; Calhoun et al. 2006).

The examination of PTSD comorbidity in clinical and epidemiologic studies has shown that persons with comorbid conditions may have more severe PTSD symptoms and be more likely to utilize mental health services (Milliken et al. 2010). For example, the cooccurrence of major depressive disorder and PTSD has been associated with poorer prognosis, greater duration and severity of illness, poorer treatment response, and higher suicide risk (Oquendo et al. 2005; Mittal et al. 2006; Campbell et al. 2007; Chan et al. 2009). Although there is a need to avoid unnecessary "labeling" of people and inadvertently contributing to the burden of mental illness, scientific studies of psychiatric comorbidity contribute to the improvement of diagnostic classification systems over time, identify possible opportunities for prevention as well as early intervention, and help to ensure that people have access to safe and effective evidence-based treatments.

REFERENCES

Acierno R, Ruggiero KJ, Galea S, et al. 2007. Psychological sequelae resulting from the 2004 Florida hurricanes: implications for postdisaster intervention. *Am J Public Health.* 97(Suppl 1):S103–S108.

Axelrod SR, Morgan CA III, Southwick SM. 2005. Symptoms of posttraumatic stress disorder and borderline personality disorder in veterans of Operation Desert Storm. *Am J Psychiatry.* 162:270–275.

Barrett DH, Resnick HS, Foy DW, et al. 1996. Combat exposure and adult psychosocial adjustment among U.S. Army veterans serving in Vietnam, 1965–1971. *J Abn Psychol.* 105:575–581.

Beckham JC, Moore SD, Feldman ME, et al. 1998. Health status, somatization, and severity of posttraumatic stress disorder in Vietnam combat veterans with posttraumatic stress disorder. *Am J Psychiatry.* 155:1565–1569.

Black DW, Blum N, Letuchy E, et al. 2006. Borderline personality disorder and traits in veterans: psychiatric comorbidity, healthcare utilization, and quality of life along a continuum of severity. *CNS Spectr.* 11:680–689.

Bollinger AR, Riggs DS, Blake DD, Ruzek JI. 2000. Prevalence of personality disorders among combat veterans with posttraumatic stress disorder. *J Trauma Stress.* 13:255–270.

Boudreaux E, Kilpatrick DG, Resnick HS, et al. 1998. Criminal victimization, posttraumatic stress disorder, and comorbid psychopathology among a community sample of women. *J Trauma Stress.* 11:665–678.

Braakman MH, Kortmann FA, van den Brink W, Verkes RJ. 2008. Post-traumatic stress disorder with secondary psychotic features: neurobiological findings. *Prog Brain Res.* 167:299–302.

Braakman MH, Kortmann FA, van den Brink W. 2009. Validity of 'post-traumatic stress disorder with secondary psychotic features': a review of the evidence. *Acta Psychiatr Scand.* 119:15–24.

Brady KT. 1997. Posttraumatic stress disorder and comorbidity: recognizing the many faces of PTSD. *J Clin Psychiatry.* 58(Suppl 9):12–15.

Brady KT, Killeen TK, Brewerton T, Lucerini S. 2000. Comorbidity of psychiatric disorders and posttraumatic stress disorder. *J Clin Psychiatry.* 61(Suppl 7):22–32.

Bryant RA. 2011. Acute stress disorder as a predictor of posttraumatic stress disorder: a systematic review. *J Clin Psychiatry.* 72:233–239.

Breslau N, Davis GC, Andreski P, Peterson E. 1991. Traumatic events and posttraumatic stress disorder in an urban population of young adults. *Arch Gen Psychiatry.* 48:216–222.

Breslau N, Davis GC. 1992. Posttraumatic stress disorder in an urban population of young adults: risk factors for chronicity. *Am J Psychiatry.* 149:671–675.

Breslau N, Davis GC, Peterson EL, Schultz L. 1997. Psychiatric sequelae of posttraumatic stress disorder in women. *Arch Gen Psychiatry.* 54:81–87.

Brewerton TD. 2007. Eating disorders, trauma, and comorbidity: focus on PTSD. *Eat Disord.* 15:285–304.

Bremner JD, Southwick SM, Johnson DR, et al. 1993. Childhood physical abuse and combat-related posttraumatic stress disorder in Vietnam veterans. *Am J Psychiatry.* 150:235–239.

Brown C, Schulberg HC, Madonia MJ, et al. 1996. Treatment outcomes for primary care patients with major depression and lifetime anxiety disorders. *Am J Psychiatry.* 153:1293–1300.

Cabrera OA, Hoge CW, Bliese PD, et al. 2007. Childhood adversity and combat as predictors of depression and post-traumatic stress in deployed troops. *Am J Prev Med.* 33:77–82.

Calhoun PS, Bosworth HB, Stechuchak KA, et al. 2006. The impact of posttraumatic stress disorder on quality of life and health service utilization among veterans who have schizophrenia. *J Trauma Stress.* 19:393–397.

Calhoun PS, Wiley M, Dennis MF, Beckham JC. 2009. Self-reported health and physician diagnosed illnesses in women with posttraumatic stress disorder and major depressive disorder. *J Traumatic Stress.* 22:122–130.

Campbell DG, Felker BL, Liu CF, et al. 2007. Prevalence of depression-PTSD comorbidity: implications for clinical practice guidelines and primary care-based interventions. *J Gen Int Med.* 22:711–718.

Chan D, Cheadle AD, Reiber G, et al. 2009. Health care utilization and its costs for depressed veterans with and without comorbid PTSD symptoms. *Psychiatric Services.* 60:1612–1617.

Classen CC, Pain C, Field NP, Woods P. 2006. Posttraumatic personality disorder: a reformulation of complex posttraumatic stress disorder and borderline personality disorder. *Psychiatr Clin North Am.* 29:87–112.

Compton WM, Conway KP, Stinson FS, et al. 2003. Prevalence, correlates, and comorbidity of DSM-IV antisocial personality syndromes and alcohol and specific drug use disorders in the United States: results from the National Epidemiologic Survey on Alcohol and Related Conditions. *J Clin Psychiatry.* 66:677–685.

Connor KM, Davidson JR, Hughes DC, et al. 2002. The impact of borderline personality disorder on post-traumatic stress in the community: a study of health status, health utilization, and functioning. *Compr Psychiatry.* 43:41–48.

Connor DF, Ford JD, Albert DB, Doerfler LA. 2007. Conduct disorder subtype and comorbidity. *Ann Clin Psychiatry.* 19:161–168.

Cougle JR, Feldner MT, Keough ME, et al. 2010. Comorbid panic attacks among individuals with posttraumatic stress disorder: associations with traumatic event exposure history, symptoms, and impairment. *J Anxiety Disord.* 24:183–188.

Creamer M, Burgess P, McFarlane AC. 2001. Post-traumatic stress disorder: findings from the Australian National Survey of Mental Health and Well-Being. *Psychol Med.* 31:1237–1247.

Crowson JJ Jr, Frueh BC, Beidel DC, Turner SM. 1998. Self-reported symptoms of social anxiety in a sample of combat veterans with posttraumatic stress disorder. *J Anxiety Disord.* 12:605–612.

Dansky BS, Brewerton TD, O'Neil PM, Kilpatrick DG. 1997. The National Women's Study: relationship of crime victimization and PTSD to bulimia nervosa. *Int J Eating Disorders.* 21:213–228.

David D, Kutcher GS, Jackson EI, Mellman TA. 1999. Psychotic symptoms in combat-related posttraumatic stress disorder. *J Clin Psychiatry.* 60:29–32.

Davidson JR, Hughes D, Blazer DG, George LK. 1991. Post-traumatic stress disorder in the community: an epidemiological study. *Psychol Med.* 21:713–721.

Dell'osso L, Carmassi C, Massimetti G, et al. 2011. Full and partial PTSD among young adult survivors 10 months after the L'Aquila 2009 earthquake: gender differences. *J Affect Disord.* 131:79–83.

Dobie DJ, Kivlahan DR, Maynard C, et al. 2004. Posttraumatic stress disorder in female veterans. Association with self-reported health problems and functional impairment. *Arch Intern Med.* 164:394–400.

Dunn NJ, Yanasak E, Schillaci J, et al. 2004. Personality disorders in veterans with posttraumatic stress disorder and depression. *J Traumatic Stress.* 17:75–82.

Engdahl B, Dikel TN, Eberly R, et al. 1998. Comorbidity and course of psychiatric disorder in a community sample of former prisoners of war. *Am J Psychiatry.* 155:1740–1745.

Engel CC, Oxman T, Yamamoto C, et al. 2008. RESPECT-Mil: feasibility of a systems-level collaborative care approach to depression and post-traumatic stress disorder in military primary care. *Mil Med.* 173:935–940.

Famularo R, Kinscherff R, Fenton T. 1991. Posttraumatic stress disorder among children clinically diagnosed as borderline personality disorder. *J Nerv Mental Dis.* 179:428–431.

Fan F, Zhang Y, Yang Y, et al. 2011. Symptoms of posttraumatic stress disorder, depression, and anxiety among adolescents following the 2008 Wenchuan earthquake in China. *J Trauma Stress*. 24:44–53.

Freeman MP, Freeman SA, McElroy SL. 2002. The comorbidity of bipolar and anxiety disorders: prevalence, psychobiology, and treatment issues. *J Affect Disord*. 68:1–623.

Friedman MJ, Resick PA, Bryant RA, Brewin CR. 2011. Considering PTSD for DSM-5. *Depress* Anxiety. 28:750–769.

Fullerton CS, Ursano RJ, Wang L. 2004. Acute stress disorder, posttraumatic stress disorder, and depression in disaster or rescue workers. *Am J Psychiatry*. 161:1370–1376.

Gershuny BS, Baer L, Parker H, et al. 2008. Trauma and posttraumatic stress disorder in treatment-resistant obsessive-compulsive disorder. *Depress Anxiety*. 25:69–71.

Gill J, Luckenbaugh D, Charney D, Vythilingam M. 2010. Sustained elevation of serum interleukin-6 and relative insensitivity to hydrocortisone differentiates posttraumatic stress disorder with and without depression. *Biol Psychiatry*. 68:999–1006.

Ginzburg K, Ein-Dor T, Solomon Z. 2010. Comorbidity of posttraumatic stress disorder, anxiety and depression: a 20-year longitudinal study of war veterans. *J Affect Disord*. 123:249–257.

Gleaves DH, Eberenz KP, May MC. 1998. Scope and significance of posttraumatic symptomatology among women hospitalized for an eating disorder. *Int J Eat Disord*. 24:147–156.

Goldstein RB, Compton WM, Grant BF. 2010. Antisocial behavioral syndromes and additional psychiatric comorbidity in posttraumatic stress disorder among U.S. adults: results from wave 2 of the National Epidemiologic Survey on Alcohol and Related Conditions. *J Am Psychiatr Nurses Assoc*. 16:145–165.

Golier JA, Yehuda R, Bierer LM, et al. 2003. The relationship of borderline personality disorder to posttraumatic stress disorder and traumatic events. *Am J Psychiatry*. 160:2018–2024.

Goodwin RD, Hamilton SP. 2003. Lifetime comorbidity of antisocial personality disorder and anxiety disorders among adults in the community. *Psychiatry Res*. 117:159–166.

Grant DM, Beck JG, Marques L, et al. 2008. The structure of distress following trauma: posttraumatic stress disorder, major depressive disorder, and generalized anxiety disorder. *J Abnorm Psychol.* 117:662–672.

Gros DF, Simms LJ, Acierno R. 2010. Specificity of posttraumatic stress disorder symptoms. An investigation of comorbidity between posttraumatic stress disorder symptoms and depression in treatment-seeking veterans. *J Nerv Men Dis.* 198:885–890.

Gunderson JG, Sabo AN. 1993. The phenomenological and conceptual interface between borderline personality disorder and PTSD. *Am J Psychiatry.* 150:19–27.

Hamner MB, Frueh BC, Ulmer HG, Arana GW. 1999. Psychotic features and illness severity in combat veterans with chronic posttraumatic stress disorder. *Biol Psychiatry.* 45:846–852.

Handley RV, Salkovskis PM, Scragg P, Ehlers A. 2009. Clinically significant avoidance of public transport following the London bombings: travel phobia or subthreshold posttraumatic stress disorder? *J Anxiety Disord.* 23:1170–1176.

Handwerger K. 2009. Differential patterns of HPA activity and reactivity in adult posttraumatic stress disorder and major depressive disorder. *Harv Rev Psychiatry.* 17:184–205.

Harned MS, Rizvi SL, Linehan MM. 2010. Impact of co-occurring posttraumatic stress disorder on suicidal women with borderline personality disorder. *Am J Psychiatry.* 167:1210–1217.

Heffernan K, Cloitre M. 2000. A comparison of posttraumatic stress disorder with and without borderline personality disorder among women with a history of childhood sexual abuse: etiological and clinical characteristics. *J Nerv Ment Dis.* 188:589–595.

Hegel MT, Unutzer J, Tang L, et al. 2005. Impact of comorbid panic and posttraumatic stress disorder on outcomes of collaborative care for late-life depression in primary care. *Am J Geriatr Psychiatry.* 13:48–58.

Helzer JE, Robins LN, McEvoy L. 1987. Post-traumatic stress disorder in the general population. *N Engl J Med.* 317:1630–1634.

Herman J, Perry JC, van der Kolk BA. 1989. Childhood trauma in borderline personality disorder. *Am J Psychiatry.* 146:490–495.

Hofmann SG, Litz BT, Weathers FW. 2003. Social anxiety, depression, and PTSD in Vietnam veterans. *J Anxiety Disord.* 17:573–582.

Hoge CW, Auchterlonie JL, Milliken CS. 2006. Mental health problems, use of mental health services, and attrition from military service after returning from deployment to Iraq or Afghanistan. *JAMA.* 295:1023–1032.

Hudziak JJ, Boffeli TJ, Kriesman JJ, et al. 1996. Clinical study of the relation of borderline personality disorder to Briquet's syndrome (hysteria), somatization disorder, antisocial personality disorder, and substance abuse disorders. *Am J Psychiatry.* 153:1598–1606.

Huppert JD, Moser JS, Gershuny BS, et al. 2005. The relationship between obsessive-compulsive and posttraumatic stress symptoms in clinical and non-clinical samples. *J Anxiety Disord.* 19:127–136.

Ikin JF, Creamer MC, Sim MR, McKenzie DP. 2010. Comorbidity of PTSD and depression in Korean War veterans: prevalence, predictors, and impairment. *J Affect Disord.* 125:279–286.

International Statistical Classification of Diseases and Related Health Problems. 2007. 10th revision. Geneva: World Health Organization.

Jacobsen LK, Southwick SM, Kosten TR. 2001. Substance use disorders in patients with posttraumatic stress disorder: a review of the literature. *Am J Psychiatry.* 158:1184–1190.

Jogems-Kosterman BJ, de Knijff DW, Kusters R, van Hoof JJ. 2007. Basal cortisol and DHEA levels in women with borderline personality disorder. *J Psychiatric Res.* 41:1019–1026.

Jordan BK, Schlenger WE, Hough R, et al. 1991. Lifetime and current prevalence of specific psychiatric disorders among Vietnam veterans and controls. *Arch Gen Psychiatry.* 48:207–215.

Kangas M, Henry JL, Bryant RA. 2005. Predictors of posttraumatic stress disorder following cancer. *Health Psychol.* 24:579–585.

Kennedy JE, Jaffee MS, Leskin GA, et al. 2007. Posttraumatic stress disorder and posttraumatic stress disorder-like symptoms and mild traumatic brain injury. *J Rehab Res Dev.* 44:895–920.

Kessler RC, Sonnega A, Bromet E, et al. 1995. Posttraumatic stress disorder in the National Comorbidity Survey. *Arch Gen Psychiatry.* 52:1048–1060.

Kessler RC, Rubinow DR, Homes C, et al. 1997. The epidemiology of DSM-III-R bipolar I disorder in a general population survey. *Psychol Med.* 27:1079–1089.

Kessler RC, Wittchen HU. 2002. Patterns and correlates of generalized anxiety disorder in community samples. *J Clin Psychiatry.* 63(Suppl 8):4–10.

Krishnan KR. 2005. Psychiatric and medical comorbidities of bipolar disorder. *Psychosomatic Med.* 67:1–8.

Lange W, Wulff H, Berea C, et al. 2005. Dexamethasone suppression test in borderline personality disorder—effects of posttraumatic stress disorder. *Psychoneuroendocrinology.* 30:919–923.

Lanius RA, Frewen PA, Girotti M, et al. 2007. Neural correlates of trauma script-imagery in posttraumatic stress disorder with and without comorbid major depression: a functional MRI investigation. *Psychiatry Res.* 155:45–56.

Laugharne J, Lillee A, Janca A. 2010. Role of psychological trauma in the cause and treatment of anxiety and depressive disorders. *Curr Opin Psychiatry.* 23:25–29.

Lee JH, Dunner DL. 2008. The effect of anxiety disorder comorbidity on treatment resistant bipolar disorders. *Depress Anxiety.* 25:91–97.

Liebschutz J, Saitz R, Brower V, et al. 2007. PTSD in urban primary care: high prevalence and low physician recognition. *J Gen Intern Med.* 22:719–726.

Lowe B, Kroenke K, Spitzer RL, et al. 2011. Trauma exposure and posttraumatic stress disorder in primary care patients: cross-sectional criterion standard study. *J Clin Psychiatry.* 72:304–312.

Luxton DD, Skopp NA, Maguen S. 2010. Gender differences in depression and PTSD symptoms following combat exposure. *Depress Anxiety.* 27:1027–1033.

Mahon J, Bradeley SN, Harvey PK, et al. 2001. Childhood trauma has dose-effect relationship with dropping out from psychotherapeutic treatment for bulimia nervosa: a replication. *Int J Eating Disorders.* 30:138–148.

Mayou R, Bryant B, Ehlers A. 2001. Prediction of psychological outcomes one year after a motor vehicle accident. *Am J Psychiatry.* 158:1231–1238.

Merikangas KR, Akiskal HS, Angst J, et al. 2007. Lifetime and 12-month prevalence of bipolar spectrum disorder in the National Comorbidity Survey Replication. *Arch Gen Psychiatry.* 64:543–552.

Milliken CS, Auchterlonie JL, Hoge CW. 2007. Longitudinal assessment of mental health problems among active and reserve component soldiers returning from the Iraq war. *JAMA.* 298:2141–2148.

Mittal D, Fortney JC, Pyne JM, et al. 2006. Impact of comorbid anxiety disorders on health-related quality of life among patients with major depressive disorder. *Psychiatric Services.* 57:1731–1737.

Mueser KT, Rosenberg SD, Goodman LA, Trumbetta SL. 2002. Trauma, PTSD, and the course of severe mental illness: an interactive model. *Schizophr Res.* 53:123–143.

Mueser KT, Salyers MP, Rosenberg SD, et al. 2004. Interpersonal trauma and posttraumatic stress disorder in patients with severe mental illness: demographic, clinical, and health correlates. *Schizophrenia bulletin.* 30:45–57.

Myer L, Smit J, Roux LL, et al. 2008. Common mental disorders among HIV-infected individuals in South Africa: prevalence, predictors, and validation of brief psychiatric rating scales. *AIDS Patient Care STDs.* 22:147–158.

Neria Y, Olfson M, Gameroff MJ, et al. 2008. Trauma exposure and posttraumatic stress disorder among primary care patients with bipolar spectrum disorder. *Bipolar Disord.* 10:503–510.

Nixon RDV, Resick PA, Nishith P. 2004. An exploration of comorbid depression among female victims of intimate partner violence with posttraumatic stress disorder. *J Affect Disord.* 82:315–320.

O'Donnell ML, Creamer M, Pattison P. 2004. Posttraumatic stress disorder and depression following trauma: understanding comorbidity. *Am J Psychiatry.* 161:1390–1396.

Ogata S, Silk KR, Goodrich S, et al. 1990. Childhood sexual and physical abuse in adult patients with borderline personality disorder. *Am J Psychiatry.* 147:1008–1013.

Oquendo M, Brent DA, Birmaher B, et al. 2005. Posttraumatic stress disorder comorbid with major depression: factors mediating the association with suicidal behavior. *Am J Psychiatry.* 162:560–566.

Olley BO, Zeier MD, Seedat S, Stein DJ. 2005. Post-traumatic stress disorder among recently diagnosed patients with HIV/AIDS in South Africa. *AIDS Care.* 17:550–557.

Orsillo SM, Heimberg RG, Juster HR, Garrett J. 1996. Social phobia and PTSD in Vietnam veterans. *J Trauma Stress.* 9:235–252.

Otto MW, Perlman CA, Wernicke R, et al. 2004. Posttraumatic stress disorder in patients with bipolar disorder: a review of prevalence, correlates, and treatment strategies. *Bipolar Disord.* 6:470–479.

Pagura J, Stein MB, Bolton JM, et al. 2010. Comorbidity of borderline personality disorder and posttraumatic stress disorder in the U.S. population. *J Psychiatr Res.* 44:1190–1198.

Picken AL, Berry K, Tarrier N, Barrowclough C. 2010. Traumatic events, posttraumatic stress disorder, attachment style, and working alliance in a sample of people with psychosis. *J Nerv Ment Dis.* 198:775–778.

Pietrzak RH, Goldstein RB, Southwick SM, Grant BF. 2010. Prevalence and Axis I comorbidity of full and partial posttraumatic stress disorder in the United States: results from Wave 2 of the National Epidemiologic Survey on Alcohol and Related Conditions. *J Anxiety Disord.* 25:456–465.

Quarantini LC, Miranda-Scippa A, Nery-Fernandes F, et al. 2010. The impact of comorbid posttraumatic stress disorder on bipolar disorder patients. *J Affect Disord.* 123:71–76.

Resnick SG, Bond GR, Mueser KT. 2003. Trauma and posttraumatic stress disorder in people with schizophrenia. *J Abnormal Psychol.* 112:415–423.

Richardson JD, Elhai JD, Pedlar DJ. 2006. Association of PTSD and depression with medical and specialist care utilization in modern peacekeeping veterans in Canada with health-related disabilities. *J Clin Psychiatry.* 67:1240–1245.

Rodriquez M, Perez V, Garcia Y. 2005. Impact of traumatic experiences and violent acts upon response to treatment of a sample of Colombian women with eating disorders. *Int J Eating Disorders.* 37:299–306.

Rosen GM, Spitzer RL, McHugh PR. 2008. Problems with the post-traumatic stress disorder diagnosis and its future in DM-V (editorial). *Br J Psychiatry.* 192:3–4.

Sautter FJ, Bissette G, Wiley J, et al. 2003. Corticotropin-releasing factor in posttraumatic stress disorder (PTSD) with secondary psychotic symptoms, nonpsychotic PTSD, and healthy control subjects. *Biol Psychiatry.* 54:1382–1388.

Sautter FJ, Brailey K, Uddo MM, et al. 1999. PTSD and comorbid psychotic disorder: comparison with veterans diagnosed with PTSD or psychotic disorder. *J Traumatic Stress.* 12:73–88.

Shaw K, McFarlane A, Bookless C. 1997. The phenomenology of traumatic reactions to psychotic illness. *J Nerv Ment Dis.* 185:434–441.

Silver JM, McAllister TW, Arciniegas DB. 2009. Depression and cognitive complaints following mild traumatic brain injury. *Am J Psychiatry.* 166:653–661.

Simoni JM, Ng MT. 2000. Trauma, coping, and depression among women with HIV/AIDS in New York City. *AIDS Care.* 12:567–580.

Smith MY, Redd WH, Peyser C, Vogl D. 1999. Post-traumatic stress disorder in cancer: a review. *Psychooncology.* 8:521–537.

Smyth JM, Heron KE, Wonderlich SA, et al. 2008. The influence of reported trauma and adverse events on eating disturbance in young adults. *In J Eat Disord.* 41:195–202.

Southwick SM, Yehuda R, Giller E. 1993. Personality disorders in treatment seeking Vietnam combat veterans with post-traumatic stress disorder. *Am J Psychiatry.* 150:1020–1023.

Southwick SM, Axelrod SR, Wang S, et al. 2003. Twenty-four-hour urine cortisol in combat veterans with PTSD and comorbid borderline personality disorder. *J Nerv Ment Dis.* 191:261–262.

Stein MB, McQuaid JR, Pedrelli P, et al. 2000. Posttraumatic stress disorder in the primary care medical setting. *Gen Hosp Psychiatry.* 22:261–269.

Stein MB, Kennedy C. 2001. Major depressive and post-traumatic stress disorder comorbidity in female victims of intimate partner violence. *J Affect Disord.* 66:133–138.

Strawn JR, Adler CM, Fleck DE, et al. 2010. Post-traumatic stress symptoms and trauma exposure in youth with first episode bipolar disorder. *Early Interv Psychiatry.* 4:169–173.

Taft CT, Resick PA, Watkins LE, Panuzio J. 2009. An investigation of posttraumatic stress disorder and depressive symptomatology among female victims of interpersonal trauma. *J Fam Violence.* 24:407–415.

Tagay S, Schlegl S, Senf W. 2010. Traumatic events, posttraumatic stress symptomatology and somatoform symptoms in eating disorder patients. *Eur Eat Disord Rev.* 18:124–132.

Vaillant GE. 1992. The beginning of wisdom is never calling a patient borderline. J *Psychotherapy Res Practice.* 1:117–134.

Yehuda R, Teicher MH, Trestman RL, et al. 1996. Cortisol regulation in posttraumatic stress disorder and major depression: a chronobiological analysis. *Biol Psychiatry.* 40:79–88.

Yen S, Shea R, Battle CL, et al. 2002. Traumatic exposure and posttraumatic stress disorder in borderline, schizotypal, avoidant and obsessive-compulsive personality disorders: findings from the collaborative longitudinal personality disorders study. *J Nerv Men Dis.* 190:510–518.

Wells TS, LeardMann CA, Fortuna SO, et al. 2010. A prospective study of depression following combat deployment in support of the wars in Iraq and Afghanistan. *Am J Public Health.* 100:90–99.

Whetten K, Reif S, Whetten R, et al. 2008. Trauma, mental health, distrust, and stigma among HIV-positive persons: implications for effective care. *Psychosomatic Med.* 70:531–538.

Widom CS. 1999. Posttraumatic stress disorder in abused and neglected children grown up. *Am J Psychiatry.* 156:1223–1229.

Wingenfeld K, Driessen M, Adam B, Hill A. 2007. Overnight urinary cortisol release in women with borderline personality disorder depends on comorbid PTSD and depressive psychopathology. *Eur Psychiatry.* 22:309–312.

Wingenfeld K, Lange W, Wulff H, et al. 2007. Stability of the dexamethasone suppression test in borderline personality disorder with and without comorbid PTSD: a one-year follow-up study. *J Clin Psychol.* 63:843–850.

Zanarini MC, Frankenburg FR, Dubo ED, et al. 1998. Axis I comorbidity of borderline personality disorder. *Am J Psychiatry.* 155:1733–1739.

Zanarini MC, Gunderson JG, Marino MG, et al. 1989. Childhood experiences of borderline patients. *Compr Psychiatry.* 30:18–25.

Zatzick DF, Marmar CR, Weiss DS, et al. 1997. Posttraumatic stress disorder and functioning and quality of life outcomes in a nationally representative sample of male Vietnam veterans. *Am J Psychiatry.* 154:1690–1695.

Zimmerman M, Mattia JI. 1999. Axis I diagnostic comorbidity and borderline personality disorder. *Compr Psychiatry.* 40:245–252.

Zlotnick C, Franklin CL, Zimmerman M. 2002. Is comorbidity of posttraumatic stress disorder and borderline personality disorder related to greater pathology and impairment? *Am J Psychiatry.* 159:1940–1943.

Zlotnick C, Johnson DM, Yen S, et al. 2003. Clinical features and impairment in women with borderline personality disorder (BPD) with posttraumatic stress disorder (PTSD), BPD without PTSD, and other personality disorders with PTSD. *J Nerv Ment Dis.* 191:706–713.

Zlotnick C, Zimmerman M, Wolfsdorf BA, Mattia JI. 2001. Gender differences in patients with posttraumatic stress disorder in a general psychiatric practice. *Am J Psychiatry.* 158:1923–1925.

4

Post-Traumatic Stress Disorder and Substance Use Disorder

Steven S. Coughlin, PhD, MPH, and Laura Herrera, MD, MPH

As detailed in the Diagnostic and Statistical Manual of Mental Disorders, substance-related disorders include disorders related to the abuse of alcohol or other drug, the side effects of a medication, and toxin exposure. Substances include alcohol, amphetamine or the similarly acting sympathomimetics, cannabis, cocaine, hallucinogens, inhalants, opioids, phencyclidine (PCP) or similarly acting arylcyclohexylamines, sedatives, hypnotics, and anxiolytics (DSM-IV-TR). Many prescribed and over-the-counter medications (for example, analgesics) can also cause substance-related disorders. The main feature of substance abuse is a maladaptive pattern of use manifested by recurrent and adverse consequences related to the repeated use of the substance or substances (DSM-IV-TR). Substance dependence includes such features as tolerance, withdrawal symptoms, or a pattern of compulsive use.

Alcohol and drug abuse and dependence are common in adolescent and adult populations in the United States and many other countries. Data about the nationwide incidence and prevalence of illicit drug and alcohol abuse and dependence among Americans aged 12 years and older are available from the National Survey on Drug Use and Health as well as from periodic surveys that focus on adolescents, college students, or specific populations (SAMHSA 2010). In 2008, an estimated 31 million people (12.4%) aged 12 or older reported driving under the influence of alcohol at least once in the past year. According to the National Survey on Drug Use and Health, current cocaine use gradually declined between 2003 and 2008 among people aged 12 or older (from 2.3 million to 1.9 million). In 2008, the number of persons aged 12 or older who abused prescription pain relievers for the first time (2.2 million) was roughly even with that of marijuana.

Surveys on illicit drug use have also been conducted among veterans and U.S. military active duty personnel. From 1980–2008, results from the Department of Defense (DoD) Health Behavior Surveys showed decreases in illicit drug use and increases in prescription drug misuse, heavy alcohol use, and post-traumatic stress disorder (PTSD; Bray et al. 2010). The prevalence of self-reported illicit drug use in the past 30 days was 5% in 2005 and 12% in 2008. Illicit drugs asked about in these anonymous DoD surveys included marijuana or hashish, cocaine, LSD, PCP, MDMA, other hallucinogens, methamphetamine, heroin, GHB/GBL, and inhalants. Prescription drugs included stimulants other than methamphetamine, tranquilizers or muscle relaxers, sedatives or barbiturates, pain relievers, and anabolic steroids. Nonmedical use of a prescription drug was defined in the surveys as any use of the drug without a doctor's prescription, in greater amounts or more often than prescribed, or for reasons such as to get "high" (Bray et al. 2010). Milliken et al. (2007) examined a variety of mental-health-related outcomes reported by soldiers returning from the Iraq War (Operation Iraqi Freedom) using data from the Post-Deployment Health Re-Assessment. About 0.2% (134 of 56,350) of active duty soldiers and 0.6% (179 of 31,885) of those in the National Guard or reserves had been referred for treatment of alcohol or substance abuse (Milliken et al. 2007). In the Iowa Gulf War Case Validation Study, which involved face-to-face interviews of 602 military personnel who had served during the time period of the first Gulf War (1990–1991), lifetime substance use disorders (including alcohol abuse or dependence) were more frequent in deployed veterans than nondeployed veterans (70% versus 52%), particularly alcohol disorders (68% versus 52%). About 21% of the deployed veterans and 20% of nondeployed veterans had a lifetime history of drug abuse or dependence.

COMORBID PTSD AND SUBSTANCE ABUSE AND DEPENDENCE OTHER THAN ALCOHOL

Clinical and epidemiologic studies have shown that substance dependence and abuse are strongly related to PTSD (Breslau and Davis 1987; Cottler et al. 1992; Mills et al. 2006; Back et al. 2009). Studies of cocaine-dependent or opioid-dependent patients (for example, those in methadone treatment programs) have found a lifetime prevalence of PTSD in the range of 10–30% (Nunes and Blanco 2009). Histories of significant trauma and PTSD are common among patients in treatment programs for substance dependence (Nunes and Blanco 2009). Department of Veterans Affairs (VA) substance use disorder treatment programs have reported rates of current PTSD as high as 35–46% (Hyer et al. 1991; Young et al. 2005). Substance use disorders are frequently seen among patients treated for PTSD (Jacobsen et al. 2001).

Reynolds et al. (2005) examined the prevalence of comorbid substance abuse disorder and PTSD in an inpatient clinical population in Great Britain. In their cross-sectional study involving chart review and interviews of substance abuse disorder patients about traumatic experiences, PTSD, and addiction, 94% of patients reported experiencing one or more PTSD criterion A traumatic experiences, 38.5% met criteria for current PTSD and 51.9% for lifetime history of PTSD (Reynolds et al. 2005).

In civilian populations, estimates of the lifetime prevalence of substance use disorders have ranged from 21.6 to 43.0% in persons with PTSD compared with 8.1–24.7% in those without PTSD (Breslau et al. 1991; Kessler et al. 1995; Jacobsen et al. 2001). Cottler et al. (1992) examined the relationship between substance abuse and PTSD in a population survey of psychiatric illness in the St. Louis Epidemiologic Catchment Area Study. Among 2,633 respondents, 430 reported a traumatic rate that could qualify for PTSD, but the overall rate of PTSD was only 1.35% (Cottler et al. 1992). Respondents who indicated that they used cocaine or opiates were over three times as likely as comparison subjects to report a traumatic event (odds ratio = 1.8, 95% confidence interval 1.5–2.3) and were more likely to meet diagnostic criteria for PTSD. Physical attack was the most frequent traumatic event reported among cocaine/opiate users (Cottler et al. 1992). Although recall bias is a possibility, findings from their cross-sectional survey suggest that civilians who use illicit substances are more likely to be exposed to traumatic events and to develop PTSD. The relationship between substance abuse disorder and PTSD was also examined in the Australian National Survey of Mental Health and Well-being (Mills et al. 2006). In a sample of 10,641 survey participants from the general population of Australia, 0.5% of the participants were found to have both PTSD and a substance use disorder (Mills et al. 2006). Individuals with comorbid substance use disorder and PTSD were found to have poorer physical and mental health and greater disability than those with a substance use disorder alone (Ouimette et al. 2006). About 61% of those with a substance use disorder and PTSD reported at least one chronic health condition compared with 35% of those with substance use disorder alone, 42% of those with PTSD alone, and 39% of those with neither disorder (Mills et al. 2006). Positive associations between PTSD and drug dependence were observed among both men and women (odds ratios 3.0 and 4.5, respectively) in the National Comorbidity Survey conducted in the United States (Kessler et al. 1995). Persons with PTSD may be relatively susceptible to opiate abuse or dependence because of the reduction in hypervigilance symptoms that these substances afford (Kosten and Krystal 1988; Young et al. 2005).

The relationship between substance abuse and PTSD has also been examined in studies of U.S. veterans. In the National Vietnam Veterans Readjustment Study, which included a cohort of 1,200 male veterans who had served in Vietnam or its surrounding waters or airspace, drug abuse or dependence was positively associated with PTSD (odds ratio = 7.4, 95% confidence interval 2.2–24.5) and with alcohol abuse or dependence (odds ratio = 3.2, 95% confidence interval 1.9–5.4; Zatzick et al. 1997). McFall et al. (1991) examined the prevalence of PTSD symptoms among Vietnam veterans treated at a Veterans Health Administration medical center substance abuse treatment facility. Of 489 male veterans presenting for treatment, about 11% had combat-related PTSD symptoms. Clinically significant PTSD symptoms occurred among 46% of the patients who had combat exposures (McFall et al. 1991). Cohen et al. (2009) examined PTSD-related conditions using national data from veterans of Operation Enduring Freedom and Operation Iraqi Freedom (OEF/OIF) who sought care at VA health care facilities. The majority of the PTSD patients in their cross-sectional study had comorbid mental health diagnoses including depression (53%), other anxiety disorder (29%), substance abuse disorder (10%), and other psychiatric diagnoses (33%). Dobie et al. (2004) surveyed women (n = 1,935) who received care at the Department of Veterans Affairs Puget Sound Health Care System between October 1996 and January 1998. The survey included questions about medical history and health habits. The PTSD Checklist-Civilian Version (PCL-C) was included. Of the 1,259 eligible women who completed the survey, 266 (21%) screened positive for current PTSD (PCL-C score ≥ 50). About 20% (51 of 253) of women with PTSD screened positive for a drug problem compared with 6% (57 of 900) of women without PTSD (age-adjusted odds ratio = 3.6, 95% confidence interval 2.4–5.4). About 31% (79 of 253) of women with PTSD screened positive for problem drinking compared with 20% (181 of 902) of women without PTSD (age-adjusted odds ratio = 1.7, 95% confidence interval 1.2–2.3). Nunnick et al. (2010) recently examined post-deployment rates of comorbid PTSD and substance abuse in a small sample (n = 36) of female veterans who served in OEF/OIF. Of the 36 participants, 11 (31%) screened positive for PTSD, 17 (47%) screened positive for high-risk drinking, and 2 (6%) screened positive for drug abuse. A positive association was observed between PTSD and higher scores on measures of alcohol and drug use ($p < 0.01$; Nunnick et al. 2010).

Longitudinal Studies of PTSD and Substance Use Disorders

The relationship between PTSD and substance abuse or dependence has been examined in relatively few longitudinal studies. Chilcoat and Breslau (1998) studied 1,007 adults aged 21 to 30 years in southeast Michigan. After an initial assessment in 1989, they were followed up three and five years later, in 1992 and 1994. Those who were found to have PTSD at the time of the initial assessment had an increased risk of drug abuse or dependence during the follow-up period (hazards ratio = 4.5, 95% confidence interval 2.6–7.6). The risk for abuse or dependence was the highest for prescribed psychoactive drugs (hazards ratio = 13.0, 95% confidence interval 5.3–32.0). Bremner et al. (1996) studied the longitudinal course of PTSD symptoms and related symptoms of alcohol and substance abuse in a sample of 61 Vietnam combat veterans with PTSD. The onset of alcohol and substance abuse was generally associated with the onset of symptoms of PTSD (Bremner et al. 1996). In addition, increases in use of alcohol and other substances paralleled the increase of PTSD symptoms. Based upon information reported by the study participants, there was a tendency for alcohol, marijuana, and benzodiazepines to improve PTSD symptoms and for cocaine to worsen symptoms in the hyperarousal category (Bremner et al. 1996).

Jacobsen et al. (2001) noted that results from published studies generally support a pathway whereby PTSD precedes substance abuse or dependence. Persons with PTSD may initially use substances to modify their symptoms. According to this "self-medication" hypothesis, persons with PTSD may use psychoactive substances to alleviate their traumatic memories and other painful symptoms (Chilcoat and Breslau 1998). Following the development of drug dependence, they may then experience distressing physiological and psychological symptoms resulting from substance withdrawal (for example, arousal symptoms that exacerbate PTSD symptoms) that contribute to a relapse of substance use (Chilcoat and Breslau 1998; Jacobsen et al. 2001). Cognitive theories of substance abuse and "tension reduction" models are also consistent with substance abuse being secondary to PTSD (Brown and Wolfe 1994). Alternative pathways may also account for linkages between PTSD and substance abuse or dependence. Some substance abusers may repeatedly place themselves in dangerous situations, and consequently be exposed to physical violence or other traumatic experiences, in the course of using or procuring illicit drugs or alcohol (Chilcoat and Breslau 1998). It is also possible that some individuals who began abusing substances at an early age may be more susceptible to developing PTSD following a traumatic exposure, because they have tended to rely on alcohol or drugs as a way to deal with stress or because of persistent changes in brain neurophysiology resulting from the abused substance (Brown and Wolfe 1994). Additional explanations such as shared vulnerability to PTSD and substance abuse following a traumatic event are also a possibility.

Longitudinal studies of PTSD and drug or alcohol use are of considerable interest in public health and medical research, partly because these comorbid conditions place persons at increased risk of HIV/AIDS and other serious health conditions (Brief et al. 2004; Drumright et al. 2006). A further issue is that in persons who are living with HIV, AIDS, or hepatitis C, comorbid conditions such as PTSD and substance abuse have important implications for adherence with treatment recommendations, quality of life, and avoidance of serious complications such as cirrhosis of the liver, adenocarcinoma of the liver, or premature mortality (Whetten et al. 2008).

ALCOHOL ABUSE AND DEPENDENCE

Alcohol is the most commonly abused brain depressant in the United States and many other countries. The main feature of alcohol abuse is a maladaptive pattern of alcohol use manifested by recurrent and adverse consequences related to the repeated use of the substance or substances (DSM-IV-TR). Alcohol dependence includes such features as tolerance, withdrawal symptoms upon cessation of use, and continued use despite persistent alcohol-related physical or psychological problems (Jacobsen et al. 2001). Physiological dependence on alcohol, with evidence of tolerance to alcohol or symptoms of withdrawal, is often associated with a more severe clinical course (DSM-IV-TR). Persons with alcohol dependence may continue to consume alcohol to avoid or reduce unpleasant withdrawal symptoms such as nausea or vomiting, autonomic hyperactivity, anxiety, and insomnia. For similar reasons, as discussed previously in the chapter, persons with PTSD may suffer from a comorbid drug disorder. Numerous studies have shown that exposure to traumatic events is associated with increased problems with alcohol use (Stewart 1996; Jacobsen et al. 2001), leading to a focused interest in the relationships between trauma, PTSD, and alcohol use disorder. A sizeable body of literature has accumulated that demonstrates that traumatic events such as sexual assault, disasters, and combat exposures can lead to alcohol abuse and dependence (Stewart 1996). In the section that follows, clinical and epidemiologic studies of comorbid PTSD, alcohol abuse, and dependence are summarized, including those that focused on clinic patients, veterans, female victims of adult sexual assault, and survivors of man-made and natural disasters.

Comorbid PTSD and Alcohol Abuse and Dependence

Studies of persons seeking treatment for alcohol dependence and population surveys have documented substantial comorbidity between PTSD and alcohol abuse and dependence. Driessen et al. (2008) studied 459 men and women who were receiving treatment at 14 addiction treatment centers in Germany. About 39.7% of the patients were receiving treatment for alcohol dependence and the remainder were receiving treatment for drug dependence (33.6%) or both alcohol and drug dependence (26.8%). About 22.5% of the patients (n = 182) receiving treatment for alcohol dependence had PTSD as compared with 39% of patients (n = 154) receiving treatment for drug dependence and 42.3% of those (n = 123) receiving treatment for both alcohol and drug dependence (Driessen et al. 2008). Studies have found that PTSD increases risk of alcohol use disorder (Stewart et al. 1999; Sonne et al. 2003). Sonne et al. (2003) examined gender differences in a sample of 84 treatment-seeking patients from the Charleston area who had comorbid PTSD and alcohol dependence. Male patients reported an earlier age of onset of alcohol dependence, greater alcohol use and craving, and more severe legal problems due to alcohol use. Female patients in this sample reported greater exposure to sexual traumas and greater social impairment due to PTSD (Sonne et al. 2003). PTSD more often preceded alcohol dependence in women than in men. Despite the small sample size and selected nature of the sample, the results from this study do suggest gender differences in comorbid PTSD and alcohol dependence. Breslau and Davis (1992) examined the frequency of alcohol abuse or dependence among 93 persons age 21 to 30 years with chronic or non-chronic PTSD who were members of a large health maintenance organization in the Detroit area. Chronic PTSD was defined as duration of PTSD symptoms of one year or more. About 36% of persons with chronic PTSD (n = 53) reported alcohol abuse or dependence as compared to 25% of those with non-chronic PTSD (adjusted OR = 2.7, 95% CI 0.9 – 7.8).

McDevitt-Murphy et al. (2010) examined associations between alcohol and drug abuse and anxiety and mood disorders in a sample of 136 college students who had been exposed to a traumatic event such as a car accident, sudden death of someone close to the respondent, sexual assault, physical assault, or assault with a weapon. The participants were assigned to one of four groups (PTSD, depression, social phobia, or well-adjusted with low levels of distress) based upon their primary diagnosis. Participants in the PTSD group reported greater alcohol consumption than those in the depressed group (McDevitt-Murphy et al. 2010). Those in the PTSD group also reported more alcohol abuse than those in the social phobia or well-adjusted groups. College students suffering from PTSD may be more likely to drink alcohol to the point of intoxication than students without PTSD, and they may also be more likely to experience subsequent traumas or to drop out of college (McDevitt-Murphy et al. 2007; Borsari et al. 2008).

The relationship between PTSD and alcohol use disorder has been examined in population surveys including the Australian National Survey of Mental Health and Well-being (Mills et al. 2006). In a sample of 10,641 survey participants from the general population of Australia, about 24% of those with PTSD had an alcohol use disorder (Mills et al. 2006). Individuals with comorbid alcohol use disorder and PTSD had poorer physical and mental health and greater disability than those with alcohol use disorder alone. Some population surveys of trauma and alcohol consumption have asked not only about frequency and level of alcohol consumption but also about patterns of use. For example, in the 2003–2004 California Women's Health Survey, a population-based, random digit dialing survey of a probability sample of women aged 18 years or older (n =

6,942), binge drinking was associated with PTSD symptoms, anxiety, and depression, as well as with adverse experiences in adulthood (for example, intimate partner violence, having been physically or sexually assaulted, or having experienced the death of someone close; Timko et al. 2008). Binge drinking was also associated with adverse experiences in childhood, such as living with someone abusing substances, mentally ill, having a mother victimized by violence, or having been physically or sexually assaulted.

Several studies have examined the relationship between PTSD and alcohol abuse and dependence among female survivors of adult sexual and physical assault (Ullman et al. 2005; Kaysen et al. 2006; Kaysen et al. 2007). Women are more likely than men to be exposed to sexual assault and chronic forms of interpersonal violence such as domestic violence or battering (Kaysen et al. 2007). Both PTSD and problem drinking are frequently observed among survivors of sexual assault, which has prompted researchers to examine whether survivors drink to cope with PTSD symptoms or whether PTSD symptoms are made worse by heavy drinking (Najdowski and Ullman 2009). Najdowski and Ullman (2009) prospectively studied an ethnically diverse sample of 555 women who were survivors of sexual assault to determine whether PTSD led to problem drinking or vice versa. Structural equation modeling was used in the analysis. The results of this study indicated that intervening sexual victimization was associated with greater symptoms of PTSD and problem drinking one year later (Najdowski and Ullman 2009). No direct influence of PTSD on problem drinking was observed, or vice versa. Kaysen et al. (2006) conducted a longitudinal study of alcohol use disorder and PTSD among female sexual (n = 69) and physical assault victims (n = 39). The participants were assessed two to four weeks and three months following their traumatic experience. Women who had a lifetime history of alcohol use disorder had higher intrusive and avoidance symptoms than those who did not have alcohol use disorder (Kaysen et al. 2006). Participants who had problems with alcohol use had the same pattern of symptom recovery as those who did not have alcohol problems but remained more symptomatic over the three months. The results of this study suggest that alcohol problems prior to trauma exposure are associated with a more severe and chronic course of PTSD symptoms among female victims of sexual or physical assault (Kaysen et al. 2006). Kaysen et al. (2007) studied alcohol use among 369 women who had been recently battered. The participants, all of whom had experienced battering within the context of an intimate relationship for three months or longer, were recruited from domestic violence shelters and other victim assistance agencies. The investigators found differences in trauma-related symptoms between abstainers, moderate drinkers, and heavy drinkers. On average, women who were heavy drinkers reported more severe symptoms (Kaysen et al. 2007). In particular, heavy drinking was associated with PTSD hyperarousal symptoms. Other studies have also found that alcohol use disorder may increase risk of developing PTSD or be associated with a more severe course of symptoms (Cottler et al. 1992; Acierno et al. 1999).

The relationship between PTSD and alcohol abuse and dependency has also been examined in veteran populations as reviewed by Stewart (1996) and others (Kulka et al. 1990; McFall et al. 1992; Jacobsen et al. 2001; Black et al. 2004; Ikin et al. 2004; Tomlinson et al. 2006; Cucciare et al. 2010; McDevitt-Murphy et al. 2010). Studies conducted in veteran populations have found that alcohol use disorders are more common among persons with PTSD than in persons not suffering from the condition (Jacobsen et al. 2001), although not all studies have shown an association between PTSD and alcohol use (Shipherd et al. 2005). In the National Vietnam Veterans Readjustment Study, about 75% of veterans with a lifetime diagnosis of PTSD met criteria for alcohol abuse or dependence (Kulka et al. 1990). McFall et al. (1992) examined the effects of Vietnam combat duty and PTSD symptoms on severity of alcohol and drug abuse disorders among 259 male Vietnam veterans treated at a Veterans Health Administration medical center substance abuse treatment facility. About 92% of the veterans presented with an alcohol abuse disorder, 60% presented with a drug abuse disorder, and 53% had both alcohol and drug abuse disorders. Veterans with PTSD experienced more severe alcohol and drug abuse problems than those without PTSD and were at higher risk for having both forms of substance abuse (McFall et al. 1992). In addition, PTSD symptomatology was more closely related to alcohol and drug abuse than level of combat exposure.

Stressful exposures that occur during wartime deployment may contribute to heavy drinking among both men and women (Brown et al. 2010; Cucciare et al. 2010; McDevitt-Murphy et al. 2010). Among male and female veterans with PTSD, alcohol abuse or dependence ranks among the most common co-morbid psychological condition. Cucciare et al. (2010) studied a sample of 554 veterans (93.5% male) who had completed a brief alcohol intervention administered by VA clinicians in outpatient settings. Veterans who were younger, used alcohol or drugs to cope with symptoms of PTSD and depression, and had experienced sexual assault, were more likely to self-report a binge drinking episode in the past 90 days. Coughlin et al. (2011) examined factors associated with alcohol use in male and female veterans of the 1990–1991 Gulf War, and in veterans who served during the same era but who were not deployed to the Gulf. Data had been collected from 9,970 respondents in 2003–2005 via a structured questionnaire or telephone survey. PTSD, major depressive disorder (MDD), unexplained multi-symptom illness (MSI), and chronic fatigue syndrome (CFS)-like illness were more frequent among veterans with problem drinking than those without problem drinking. About 28% of Gulf War veterans with problem drinking had PTSD as compared with 12.7% of Gulf War veterans without problem drinking. In multivariate analysis, problem drinking was positively associated with PTSD, MDD, unexplained MSI, and CFS-like illness after adjustment for age, sex, race, ethnicity, branch of service, rank, and Gulf status. In the model for PTSD, the adjusted odds ratio for problem drinking was 2.7 (95% confidence interval 2.3–3.2). The study was limited by its cross-sectional design and reliance on the PCL screening test for PTSD rather than clinical interviews. McDevitt-Murphy et al. (2010) examined whether alcohol abuse may mediate the relationship between PTSD and functional health outcomes in a sample of 151 OEF/OIF veterans seen at a VA primary care clinic. The participants included 136 men and 15 women. About 39.1% of the veterans screened positive for PTSD and 26.5% screened positive for hazardous drinking. Hazardous drinking was found to partially mediate the relationship between PTSD and functional mental health (McDevitt-Murphy et al. 2010). The study was limited by its cross-sectional design and by the absence of an interview-based measure of PTSD or information from participants' medical records. Seal et al. (2011) examined the prevalence and correlates of alcohol abuse and dependence (alcohol use disorder) diagnoses in OEF/OIF veterans (n = 456,502) who were new users of Department of Veterans Affairs health care between October 15, 2001, and September 30, 2009, and followed through January 1, 2010. The investigators used VA administrative data to determine the prevalence and correlates of alcohol use disorder and drug use disorder in a nationwide sample of veterans. Over 11% of the veterans in the sample had received a substance use disorder diagnosis (alcohol use disorder, drug use disorder, or both). About 10% had received an alcohol use disorder diagnosis. Of those veterans who had received a substance use disorder diagnosis, 55–75% also received PTSD or depression diagnoses, that is, post-deployment substance use disorder diagnoses were highly comorbid with PTSD and depression (Seal et al. 2011).

In addition to sexual and physical assault victims and veterans exposed to combat, the relationship between PTSD and alcohol abuse and dependence has been studied in disaster survivors (North et al. 2002; Grieger et al. 2003; Schroeder and Polusny 2004; Kohn et al. 2005; Adams et al. 2006). Studies have shown that survivors of natural and man-made disasters such as hurricanes, floods, and terrorist attacks often increase their alcohol use following the disaster (Vlahov et al. 2002; Kohn et al. 2005). Adams et al. (2006) prospectively studied a panel of adults living in New York City on the day of the terrorist attacks on the World Trade Center. A total of 2,368 persons completed the initial survey one year after the attacks, and 1,681 completed the second survey two years after the attacks. About 10% of the participants reported an increase in the amount of alcohol they consumed after the attacks compared to before the attacks (Adams et al. 2006). The outcomes examined in the study included measures of subsyndromal PTSD, partial PTSD, and depression, based upon self-reported information. The investigators examined subsyndromal and partial PTSD because the number of participants with full PTSD in this sample was relatively small. Binge drinking was found to be related to partial PTSD in multivariate analysis (Adams et al. 2006). In addition, alcohol dependence was related to subsyndromal PTSD, PTSD symptom severity, and depression. Grieger et al. (2003) examined PTSD and alcohol use in a sample of survivors of the September 11, 2001, terrorist attack on the Pentagon. The attack resulted in the death of 125 military and civilian Pentagon employees and 64 passengers and crew aboard the hijacked jet. The investigators contacted about 680 military and civilian staff in one of the Pentagon commands by electronic questionnaire; they received 77 anonymous responses via an Internet server. Of the persons who responded, 59 (77%) were men and 60 (77%) were active duty military personnel. Ten respondents (13%) reported that they had used more alcohol than they intended since September 11 (Grieger et al. 2003). Women were 6.8 times more likely than men to report increased alcohol use ($p = 0.008$, 95% confidence interval = 1.7–27.7). Persons with PTSD were 5.6 times more likely than those without PTSD to report increased alcohol use ($p = 0.023$, 95% confidence interval = 1.3–24.9).

Kohn et al. (2005) interviewed 800 persons age 15 and older in Tegucigalpa, Honduras, two months after Hurricane Mitch had caused destruction in the area. The participants were selected from residential areas of high, middle, or low socioeconomic status that had suffered either high or low impact from the devastating effects of the hurricane. Respondents from high-impact residential areas were more distressed and had greater severity of PTSD symptoms (Kohn et al. 2005). In addition, respondents from high-impact residential areas had higher prevalence rates of alcoholism and major depression. Predictors of PTSD in this sample of natural disaster survivors included degree of exposure based upon reported traumatic events. Among those with PTSD, women and those with a higher degree of exposure to hurricane-related traumatic events had a greater severity of PTSD on average (Kohn et al. 2005).

Psychological hypotheses about the relationship between alcohol abuse and PTSD often posit that PTSD precedes the development of alcohol abuse (Jacobsen et al. 2001; Coughlin et al. 2011). According to this hypothesis, alcohol problems may occur as a consequence of PTSD (McLeod et al. 2001). Persons suffering from PTSD symptoms may be more likely to use alcohol or other substances, which may in turn place them at risk of experiencing further traumatic events such as physical injury or sexual assault (Borsari et al. 2008). Like with illicit drug abuse, excessive alcohol consumption and alcohol dependence may result from attempts to "self-medicate" or alleviate disturbing memories or other symptoms associated with PTSD. For example, persons suffering from PTSD may use alcohol to reduce negative affect or hyperarousal symptoms or in an attempt to alleviate sleep difficulties (Stewart et al. 2000; Kaysen et al. 2007). Anxiety experienced during alcohol withdrawal (which may be intensified by repeated experiences of withdrawal) promotes drinking and relapse behavior (Spanagel 2009). According to the self-medication hypothesis, alcohol is used to reduce or cope with symptoms of PTSD, and alcohol use is then maintained by negative reinforcement (Kaysen et al. 2007). An alternative hypothesis is that shared stressors such as sexual assault or war-time traumas independently lead to both PTSD and problem drinking. This latter possibility has sometimes been referred to as the "shared stressor hypothesis" (McLeod et al. 2001).

Psychosocial and Medical Consequences of Comorbid PTSD and Alcohol Dependence

The co-occurrence of PTSD and alcohol use disorder has been associated with worse outcomes for both disorders. Persons with comorbid PTSD and alcohol dependence often face other challenges such as difficulties with employment, schooling, or relationships, and they may suffer from other health conditions (for example, depression or drug dependency). Alcohol dependence, with or without comorbid PTSD, can adversely affect the life of the user including loss of partner and friends, job loss, and difficulties with the legal system (Spanagel 2009). Alcohol craving and compulsive use occur and, among those who go into remission, relapses can occur even after years of abstinence (Spanagel 2009). Chronic intake of high amounts of alcohol can have adverse effects on several organ systems including the peripheral and central nervous system, and lead to cognitive deficits and memory impairment (DSM-IV-TR). Heavy alcohol use is associated with increased risk of several acute and chronic adverse health conditions including injuries, cirrhosis of the liver and other gastrointestinal illnesses, hypertension, coronary heart disease, stroke, and certain types of cancer (Rehm et al. 2003; Corrao et al. 2004). As mentioned earlier in this chapter, persons suffering from comorbid PTSD and substance abuse or dependence may also have an increased risk of HIV, AIDS, chronic hepatitis, or difficulty with treatment adherence (Brief et al. 2004).

NEUROBIOLOGY OF STRESS AND ADDICTION

The role of traumatic exposures in the etiology of anxiety and substance use disorders has been further clarified by animal studies and neurobiological research (Jacobsen et al. 2001; Nuenes and Blanco 2009). The neurobiology of addiction is complex and includes the desensitization of the brain reward system over time (Nuenes and Blanco 2009). The brain reward system is blunted after chronic drug administration. In neuroimaging studies of alcohol- and drug-dependent patients, deficits in the brain dopamine system have been shown including decreased density of dopamine D_2 receptors and decreased release of dopamine in response to dopamine-releasing drugs (Martinez et al. 2007). Another aspect of the neurobiology of addiction is drug or alcohol craving or cue-elicited drug seeking (Nuenes and Blanco 2009). Neuroimaging studies show that drug or alcohol cues activate brain regions associated with the brain reward system. Dysregulation of the hypothalamic-pituitary-adrenal (HPA) axis and corticotrophin-releasing factor (CRH) have been implicated in both PTSD and drug abuse (Jacobsen et al. 2001; Nuenes and Blanco 2009). Neurobiological research has shown that both PTSD and substance withdrawal may result in elevated levels of CRF in the brain (Jacobsen et al. 2001).

GENETICS OF PTSD AND SUBSTANCE DEPENDENCE

Alcohol use disorders are the results of cumulative responses to alcohol exposure, the genetic make-up of an individual, and environmental exposures over time (Spanagel 2009). Based upon family studies and twin studies, an estimated 40–60% of the variance of risk of alcohol dependence is explained by genetic influences (DSM-IV-TR). Results from twin studies have suggested that comorbid PTSD and alcohol dependence may be partly due to overlapping genetic influences (Xian et al. 2000; Sartor et al. 2010). Xian et al. (2000) examined the degree to which genetic environmental contributions to PTSD, alcohol dependence, and drug dependence overlap in a sample of 3,304 monozygotic and dizygotic male-male twin pairs who were identified through the Vietnam Era Twin Registry. The investigators fit genetic models to estimate genetic and environmental contributions to the lifetime co-occurrence of PTSD, alcohol dependence, and drug dependence. Risk for PTSD was partly due to a 15% genetic contribution common to alcohol dependence and drug dependence and a 20% genetic contribution specific to PTSD (Xian et al. 2000). Risk for alcohol disorder was partly due to a 56% genetic contribution shared by PTSD and drug dependence (Xian et al. 2000). Sartor et al. (2010) studied a sample of 3,768 all-female twins ranging in age from 18 to 29 years. In order to estimate genetic and environmental contributions to PTSD and the extent to which they overlap with those of alcohol dependence, the researchers fitted a trivariate genetic model that included trauma exposure as a separate phenotype. Genetic influences accounted for 72% of the variance in PTSD. Individual-specific environmental influences accounted for about 28% of the variance in PTSD. The genetic correlation between PTSD and alcohol disorder was 0.54, meaning that there was substantial overlap in genetic influences on PTSD and alcohol dependence (Sartor et al. 2010). Other studies have identified genetic and environmental influences for PTSD that are familial in nature (Breslau and Davis 1992).

CLINICAL RESEARCH QUESTIONS RELATED TO THE DUAL DIAGNOSIS OF PTSD AND SUBSTANCE USE DISORDER

Providers who care for patients with alcohol or drug use disorders and PTSD have reported that comorbid substance use disorder and PTSD are particularly challenging to treat (Back et al. 2009). The co-occurrence of a substance use disorder and PTSD in the same patient can result in a more complicated clinical presentation, higher relapse rates, more interpersonal problems, and poorer attendance at aftercare activities (Jacobsen et al. 2001; Ouimette et al. 2006; Back et al. 2009). Clinical studies indicate that patients with a substance use disorder and PTSD tend to have worse outcomes following treatment than those with a substance use disorder and no PTSD (Ouimette et al. 1997; Young et al. 2005). In addition, persons with both PTSD and a substance use disorder have been reported to have more severe PTSD symptoms as compared with persons with PTSD alone (Saladin et al. 1995; Jacobsen et al. 2001). Many patients with a comorbid substance use disorder and PTSD may only receive treatment for alcohol or drug use (or both), even though this may be contrary to patient preferences (Young et al. 2005; Back et al. 2009). Dual diagnosis treatment programs for PTSD and substance use disorder are increasingly being developed and utilized (Gulliver and Steffen 2010). In an article published in 1994, Brown and Wolfe pointed to the need for more empirical research to guide dual diagnosis treatment for PTSD and substance abuse, including studies aimed at gaining a better understanding of treatment outcomes when treatment for substance abuse and PTSD is provided simultaneously or sequentially. In the simultaneous or concurrent approach, treatment of both PTSD and substance abuse is provided early in the recovery process. In the sequential approach, a patient receives treatment for substance abuse first in order to achieve a period of sobriety before beginning treatment for PTSD (Brown and Wolfe 1994). Various approaches for treatment of patients with dual diagnosis of PTSD and substance abuse disorder, including areas for additional clinical research using randomized controlled trials, have recently been reviewed by Gulliver and Steffen (2010).

SUMMARY AND CONCLUSIONS

Studies have found that PTSD increases risk of substance use disorder including alcohol dependence (Stewart et al. 1999; Sonne et al. 2003). In addition, results from several studies indicate that substance use disorder may increase risk of developing PTSD or be associated with a more severe course of symptoms (Cottler et al. 1992; Acierno et al.1999; Kaysen et al. 2006, 2007). Persons with alcohol use disorder may experience greater avoidance and hyperarousal symptoms and more reexperiencing symptoms (Stewart et al.

1998; Read et al. 2004; Kaysen et al. 2006). In persons with comorbid PTSD and alcohol dependence, PTSD symptoms tend to be more severe, and these persons may be more susceptible to alcohol use relapse (McCarthy and Petrakis 2010). Substance abuse may contribute to the maintenance of PTSD by interfering with psychological mechanisms of processing traumatic experience or by preventing desensitization to traumatic events (Stewart 1996). Comorbid PTSD and alcohol or drug dependence may be associated with more frequent psychosocial and medical complications than either disorder alone. Dual diagnosis treatment programs for PTSD and substance use disorder are increasingly being developed and utilized; additional clinical trials of their effectiveness are likely to be conducted (Gulliver and Steffen 2010). Ongoing research in this area offers hope to persons suffering from comorbid PTSD and substance abuse or dependence.

REFERENCES

Acierno R, Resnick H, Kilpatrick DG, et al. 1999. Risk factors for rape, physical assault, and post-traumatic stress disorder in women: examination of differential multivariate relationships. *J Anxiety Disorders.* 13:541–563.

Adams RE, Boscarino JA, Galea S. 2006. Alcohol use, mental health status and psychological well-being 2 years after the World Trade Center attacks in New York City. *Am J Drug Alcohol Abuse.* 32:203–224.

Arch JJ, Craske MG, Stein MB, et al. 2006. Correlates of alcohol use among anxious and depressed primary care patients. *Gen Hosp Psychiatry.* 28:37–42.

Back SE, Waldrop AE, Brady KT. 2009. Treatment challenges associated with comorbid substance use and posttraumatic stress disorder: clinicians' perspectives. *Am J Addict.* 18:15–20.

Black DW, Carney CP, Forman-Hoffman VL, et al. 2004. Depression in veterans of the first Gulf War and comparable military controls. *Ann Clin Psychiatry.* 16:53–61.

Bleich A, Gelkopf M, Solomon Z. 2003. Exposure to terrorism, stress-related mental health symptoms, and coping behaviors among a nationally representative sample in Israel. *JAMA.* 290:612–620.

Borsari B, Read JP, Campbell JF. 2008. Posttraumatic stress disorder and substance use disorders in college students. *J College Stud Psychother.* 22:61–85.

Boscarino JA, Adams RE, Galea S. 2006. Alcohol use in New York after the terrorist attacks: a study of the effects of psychological trauma on drinking behavior. *Addict Behav.* 31:606–621.

Bray RM, Pemberton MR, Lane ME, et al. 2010. Substance use and mental health trends among U.S. military active duty personnel: key findings from the 2008 DoD Health Behavior Survey. *Mil Med.* 175:390–399.

Bremner JD, Southwick SM, Darnell A, Charney DS. 1996. Chronic PTSD in Vietnam combat veterans: course of illness and substance abuse. *Am J Psychiatry.* 153:369–375.

Breslau N, Davis GC. 1987. Posttraumatic stress disorder: the etiologic specificity of wartime stressors. *Am J Psychiatry.* 144:578–583.

Breslau N, Davis GC. 1992. Posttraumatic stress disorder in an urban population of young adults: risk factors for chronicity. *Am J Psychiatry.* 149:671–675.

Breslau N, Davis GC, Andreski P, Peterson E. 1991. Traumatic events and posttraumatic stress disorder in an urban population of young adults. *Arch Gen Psychiatry.* 48:216–222.

Bridevaux IP, Bradley KA, Bryson CL, et al. 2004. Alcohol screening results in elderly male veterans: association with health status and mortality. *J Am Geriatr Soc.* 52:1510–1517.

Brief DJ, Bollinger AR, Vielhauer MJ, et al. 2004. Understanding the interface of HIV, trauma, post-traumatic stress disorder, and substance use and its implications for health outcomes. *AIDS Care.* 16(Suppl 1):S97–S120.

Brown JM, Bray RM, Hartzell MC. 2010. A comparison of alcohol use and related problems among women and men in the military. *Mil Med.* 175:101–107.

Brown PJ, Wolfe J. 1994. Substance abuse and post-traumatic stress disorder comorbidity. *Drug and Alcohol Dependence.* 35:51–59.

Chilcoat HD, Breslau N. 1998. Posttraumatic stress disorder and drug disorders: testing causal pathways. *Arch Gen Psychiatry.* 55:913–917.

Cohen BE, Marmar C, Ren L, et al. 2009. Association of cardiovascular risk factors with mental health diagnoses in Iraq and Afghanistan War Veterans using VA health care. *JAMA.* 302:489–492.

Corrao G, Bagnardi V, Zambon A, La Vecchia C. 2004. A meta-analysis of alcohol consumption and the risk of 15 diseases. *Prev Med.* 38:613–619.

Cottler LB, Compton WM, Mager D, et al. 1992. Posttraumatic stress disorder among substance users from the general population. *Am J Psychiatry.* 149:664–670.

Coughlin SS, Kang HK, Mahan CM. 2011. Alcohol use and selected health conditions in veterans who served in the 1991 Gulf War: results from a survey conducted 12 to 14 years after the war. *Prev Chronic Dis.* 8(3). Avaliable at:http://www.cdc.gov/pcd/issues/2011/may/10_0164.htm. Accessed January 4, 2012.

Cucciare MA, Darrow M, Weingardt KR. 2011. Characterizing binge drinking among U.S. military veterans receiving a brief alcohol intervention. *Addictive Behaviors.* 36:362–367.

Del Boca FK, Darkes J. 2003. The validity of self-reports of alcohol consumption: state of the science and challenges for research. *Addiction.* 98(Suppl 2):1–12.

Dobie DJ, Kivlahan DR, Maynard C, et al. 2004. Posttraumatic stress disorder in female veterans. Association with self-reported health problems and functional impairment. *Arch Intern Med.* 164:394–400.

Driessen M, Schulte S, Luedecke C, et al. 2008. Trauma and PTSD in patients with alcohol, drug, or dual dependence: a multi-center study. *Alcohol Clin Exp Res.* 32:481–488.

Drumright LN, Little SJ, Strathdee SA, et al. 2006. Unprotected anal intercourse and substance use among men who have sex with men with recent HIV infection. *J Acquir Immune Defic Syndr.* 43:344–350.

Eisen SA, Kang HK, Murphy FM, et al. 2005. Gulf War Veterans' health: medical evaluation of a U.S. cohort. *Ann Intern Med.* 142:881–890.

Gray GC, Coate BD, Anderson CH, et al. 1996. The postwar hospitalization experience of U.S. Veterans of the Persian Gulf War. *N Engl J Med.* 335:1505–1513.

Grieger TA, Fullerton CS, Urasano RJ. 2003. Posttraumatic stress disorder, alcohol use, and perceived safety after the terrorist attack on the Pentagon. *Psychiatric Services.* 54:1380–1382.

Gulliver SB, Steffen LE. 2010. Towards integrated treatments for PTSD and substance use disorders. *PTSD Research Quarterly.* 21:1–7.

Hawkins EJ, Lapham GT, Kivlahan DR, Bradley KA. 2010. Recognition and management of alcohol misuse in OEF/OIF and other veterans in the VA: a cross-sectional study. *Drug Alcohol Depend.* 109:147–153.

Hedges DW, Woon FL. 2010. Alcohol use and hippocampal volume deficits in adults with posttraumatic stress disorder: a meta-analysis. *Biol Psychol.* 84:163–168.

Hyer L, Leach P, Boudewyns PA, Davis H. 1991. Hidden PTSD in substance abuse inpatients among Vietnam veterans. *J Substance Abuse Treatment.* 8:213–219.

Ikin JF, Sim MR, Creamer MC, et al. 2004. War-related psychological stressors and risk of psychological disorders in Australian veterans of the 1991 Gulf War. *Br J Psychiatry.* 185:116–126.

Iversen A, Waterdrinker A, Fear N, et al. 2007. Factors associated with heavy alcohol consumption in the U.K. armed forces: data from a health survey of Gulf, Bosnia, and era veterans. *Mil Med.* 172:956–961.

Jacobsen LK, Southwick SM, Kosten TR. 2001. Substance use disorders in patients with posttraumatic stress disorder: a review of the literature. *Am J Psychiatry.* 158:1184–1190.

Kaysen D, Simpson T, Dillworth T, et al. 2006. Alcohol problems and posttraumatic stress disorder in female crime victims. *J Trauma Stress.* 19:399–403.

Kaysen D, Dillworth TM, Simpson T, et al. 2007. Domestic violence and alcohol use: trauma-related symptoms and motives for drinking. *Addict Behav.* 32:1272–1283.

Kaysen D, Pantalone DW, Chawla N, et al. 2008. Posttraumatic stress disorder, alcohol use, and physical health concerns. *J Behav Med.* 31:115–125.

Kessler RC, Sonnega A, Bromet E, Nelson CB. 1995. Posttraumatic stress disorder in the National Comorbidity Survey. *Arch Gen Psychiatry.* 52:1048–1060.

Kofoed L, Friedman MJ, Peck R. 1993. Alcoholism and drug abuse in patients with PTSD. *Psychiatric Quarterly.* 64:151–171.

Kohn R, Levav I, Donaire I, et al. 2005. Psychological and psychopathological reactions in Honduras following Hurricane Mitch: implications for service planning. *Rev Panam Salud Publica.* 18:287–295.

Kosten TR, Krystal J. 1988. Biological mechanisms in posttraumatic stress disorder: relevance for substance abuse. In: M. Galanter, editor. Recent Developments in Alcoholism. Vol. 6. New York: Plenum, 49–68.

Kulka RA, Schlenger WE, Fairbank JA, et al. 1990. Trauma and the Vietnam War generation: report of findings from the National Vietnam Veterans Readjustment Study. New York: Bruner-Mazel, 117–126.

Maguen S, Metzler TJ, McCaslin SE, et al. 2009. Routine work environment stress and PTSD symptoms in police officers. *J Nerv Ment Dis.* 197:754–760.

Martinez D, Narendran R, Foltin RW et al. 2007. Amphetamine-induced dopamine release: markedly blunted in cocaine dependence and predictive of the choice to self-administer cocaine. *Am J Psychiatry.* 164:622–629.

McCarthy E, Petrakis I. 2010. Epidemiology and management of alcohol dependence in individuals with post-traumatic stress disorder. *CNS Drugs.* 24:997–1007.

McDevitt-Murphy ME, Williams JL, Bracken KL, et al. 2010. PTSD symptoms, hazardous drinking, and health functioning among U.S. OEF and OIF veterans presenting to primary care. *J Traumatic Stress.* 23:108–111.

McDevitt-Murphy ME, Murphy JG, Monahan CJ, et al. 2010. Unique patterns of substance misuse associated with PTSD, depression, and social phobia. *J Dual Diagnosis.* 6:94–110.

McDevitt-Murphy ME, Weathers FW, Flood AM, et al. 2007. The utility of the PAI and the MMPI-2 for discriminating PTSD, depression, and social phobia in trauma-exposed college students. *Assessment.* 14:181–195.

McFall ME, Mackay PW, Donovan DM. 1991. Combat-related PTSD and psychosocial adjustment problems among substance abusing veterans. *J Nerv Ment Dis.* 179:33–38.

McFall ME, Mackay PW, Donovan DM. 1992. Combat-related posttraumatic stress disorder and severity of substance abuse in Vietnam veterans. *J Studies Alcohol.* 53:357–363.

McKenzie DP, McFarlane AC, Creamer M, et al. 2006. Hazardous or harmful alcohol use in Royal Australian Navy veterans of the 1991 Gulf War: identification of high risk subgroups. *Addict Behav.* 31:1683–694.

McLeod DS, Koenen KC, Meyer JM, et al. 2001. Genetic and environmental influences on the relationship among combat exposure, posttraumatic stress disorder symptoms, and alcohol use. *J Traumatic Stress.* 14:259–275.

Mills KL, Teesson M, Ross J, Peters L. 2006. Trauma, PTSD, and substance abuse disorders: findings from the Australian National Survey of Mental Health and Well-being. *Am J Psychiatry.* 163:651–658.

Najdowski CJ, Ullman SE. 2009. Prospective effects of sexual victimization on PTSD and problem drinking. *Addict Behav.* 34:965–968.

North CS, Tivis L, McMillen JC, et al. 2002. Psychiatric disorders in rescue workers after the Oklahoma City bombing. *Am J Psychiatry.* 159:857–859.

North CS, Pfefferbaum B, Narayanan P, et al. 2005. Comparison of post-disaster psychiatric disorders after terrorist bombings in Nairobi and Oklahoma City. *Br J Psychiatry.* 186:487–493.

Nunes EV, Blanco C. Anxiety and substance abuse. 2009. Implications for pathophysiology and DSM-V. In: Andrews G, Charney DS, Sirovatka PJ, Regier DA, editors. *Stress-Induced and Fear Circuitry Disorders. Advancing the Research Agenda for DSM-V.* Arlington, VA: American Psychiatric Association.

Nunnink SE, Goldwaser G, Heppner PS, et al. 2010. Female veterans of the OEF/OIF conflict: concordance of PTSD symptoms and substance misuse. *Addictive Behaviors.* 35:655–659.

Ouimette P, Goodwin E, Brown PJ. 2006. Health and well being of substance use disorder patients with and without posttraumatic stress disorder. *Addict Behav.* 31:1415–1423.

Ouimette PC, Ahrens C, Moos RH, Finney JW. 1997. Posttraumatic stress disorder in substance abuse patients: relationships to 1-year posttreatment outcomes. Psychology of *Addictive Behaviors.* 11:34–47.

Ray LA, Capone C, Sheets E, et al. 2009. Posttraumatic stress disorder with and without alcohol use disorders: diagnostic and clinical correlates in a psychiatric sample. *Psychiatry Res.* 170:278–281.

Read JP, Brown PJ, Kahler CW. 2004. Substance use and posttraumatic stress disorders: symptom interplay and effects on outcome. *Addictive Behaviors.* 29:1665–672.

Regier DA, Farmer ME, Rae DS, et al. 1990. Comorbidity of mental disorders with alcohol and other drug abuse. Results from the Epidemiologic Catchment Area (ECA) Study. *JAMA.* 264:2511–2518.

Rehm J, Gmel G, Sempost CT, Trevisan M. 2003. Alcohol-related morbidity and mortality. *Alcohol Research Health.* 27:39–51.

Reynolds M, Mezey G, Chapman M, et al. 2005. Co-morbid post-traumatic stress disorder in a substance misusing clinical population. *Drug Alcohol Depend.* 77:251–258.

Richman JA, Shannon CA, Rospenda KM, et al. 2009. The relationship between terrorism and distress and drinking: two years after September 11, 2001. *Subst Use Misuse.* 44:1665–1680.

Saladin ME, Brady KT, Dansky BS, Kilpatrick DG. 1995. Understanding comorbidity between PTSD and substance use disorders: two preliminary investigations. *Addict Behav.* 20:643–655.

Sartor CE, McCutcheon VV, Pommer NE, et al. 2011. Common genetic and environmental contributions to post-traumatic stress disorder and alcohol dependence in young women. *Psychol Med.* 41:1497–1505.

Scherrer JF, Xian H, Lyons MJ, et al. 2008. Posttraumatic stress disorder; combat exposure; and nicotine dependence, alcohol dependence, and major depression in male twins. *Compr Psychiatry.* 49:297–304.

Schroeder JM, Polusny MA. 2004. Risk factors for adolescent alcohol use following a natural disaster. *Prehosp Disaster Med.* 19:122–127.

Seal KH, Cohen G, Waldrop A, et al. 2011. Substance use disorders in Iraq and Afghanistan veterans in VA healthcare, 2001-2010: implications for screening, diagnosis and treatment. *Drug Alcohol Depend.* 116:93–101.

Shipherd JC, Stafford J, Tanner LR. 2005. Predicting alcohol and drug abuse in Persian Gulf War veterans: what role do PTSD symptoms play? *Addictive Behaviors.* 30:595–599.

Sonne SC, Back SE, Diaz Zuniga C, et al. 2003. Gender differences in individuals with comorbid alcohol dependence and post-traumatic stress disorder. *Am J Addict.* 12:412–423.

Spanagel R. 2009. Alcoholism: a systems approach from molecular physiology to addictive behavior. *Physiol Rev.* 89:649–705.

Spoont MR, Murdoch M, Hodges J, et al. 2010. Treatment receipt by Veterans after a PTSD diagnosis in PTSD, mental health, or general medical clinics. *Psychiatric Services.* 61:58–63.

Stahre MA, Brewer RD, Fonseca VP, Naimi TS. 2009. Binge drinking among U.S. active-duty military personnel. *Am J Prev Med.* 36:208–217.

Stewart SH, Conrod PJ, Pihl RO, Dongier M. 1999. Relations between posttraumatic stress symptom dimensions and substance dependence in a community-recruited sample of substance abusing women. *Psychology of Addictive Behaviors.* 13:78–88.

Stewart SH, Conrod PJ, Samoluk SB, et al. 2000. Posttraumatic stress disorder symptoms and situation-specific drinking in women substance abusers. *Alcoholism Treatment Quarterly*. 18:31–47.

Stewart SH, Mitchell TL, Wright KD, Loba P. 2004. The relations of PTSD symptoms to alcohol use and coping drinking in volunteers who responded to the Swissair Flight 111 airline disaster. *J Anxiety Disord*. 18:51–68.

Stewart SH. 1996. Alcohol abuse in individuals exposed to trauma: a critical review. *Psychological Bulletin*. 120:83–112.

Stimpson NJ, Thomas HV, Weightman AL, et al. 2003. Psychiatric disorders in veterans of the Persian Gulf War of 1991. *Br J Psychiatry*. 182:391–403.

Substance Abuse and Mental Health Services Administration, Office of Applied Studies Avaliable at: http://oas.samhsa.gov/NSDUHLatest.htm. Accessed January 4, 2012.

Taft CT, Kaloupek DG, Schumm JA, et al. 2007. Posttraumatic stress disorder symptoms, physiological reactivity, alcohol problems, and aggression among military veterans. *J Abnorm Psychol*. 116:498–507.

Timko C, Sutkowi A, Pavao J, Kimerling R. 2008. Women's childhood and adult adverse experiences, mental health, and binge drinking; the California Women's Health Survey. *Substance Abuse Treatment Prev Policy*. 3:15, Avaliable at:http://www.substanceabusepolicy.com/content/3/1/15. Accessed January 4, 2012.

Tomlinson KL, Tate SR, Anderson KG, et al. 2006. An examination of self-medication and rebound effects: psychiatric symptomatology before and after alcohol or drug relapse. *Addictive Behaviors*. 31:461–474.

Toomey R, Kang HK, Karlinsky J, et al. 2007. Mental health of US Gulf War veterans 10 years after the war. *Br J Psychiatry*. 190:385–393.

Ullman SE, Filipas HH, Townsend SM, Starzynski LL. Ullman SE, Filipas HH, Townsend SM, Starzynski LL. 2005. Trauma exposure, posttraumatic stress disorder and problem drinking in sexual assault survivors. *J Stud Alcohol*. 66:610–619.

Vlahov D, Galea S, Ahern J, et al. 2004. Consumption of cigarettes, alcohol, and marijuana among New York City residents six months after the September 11 terrorist attacks. *Am J Drug Alcohol Abuse*. 30:385–407.

Waldrop AE, Back SE, Sensenig A, Brady KT. 2008. Sleep disturbances associated with posttraumatic stress disorder and alcohol dependence. *Addict Behav*. 33:328–335.

Whetten K, Reif S, Whetten R, Murphy-McMillan LK. 2008. Trauma, mental health, distrust, and stigma among HIV-positive presons: implications for effective care. *Psychosomatic Med.* 70:531–538.

Wilk JE, Bliese PD, Kim PY, et al. 2010. Relationship of combat experiences to alcohol misuse among U.S. soldiers returning from the Iraq war. *Drug Alcohol Depend.* 108:115–121.

Woodward SH, Kaloupek DG, Streeter CC, et al. 2006. Hippocampal volume, PTSD, and alcoholism in combat veterans. *Am J Psychiatry.* 163:674–681.

Xian H, Chantarujikapong SI, Scherrer JF, et al. 2000. Genetic and environmental influences on posttraumatic stress disorder, alcohol and drug dependence in twin pairs. *Drug Alcohol Dep.* 61:95–102.

Xian H, Scherrer JF, Grant JD, et al. 2008. Genetic and environmental contributions to nicotine, alcohol and cannabis dependence in male twins. *Addiction.* 103:1391–1398.

Young HE, Rosen CS, Finney JW. 2005. A survey of PTSD screening and referral practices in VA addiction treatment programs. *J Subst Abuse Treat.* 28:313–319.

Zatzick DF, Marmar CR, Weiss DS, et al. 1997. Posttraumatic stress disorder and functioning and quality of life outcomes in a Nationally Representative Sample of Male Vietnam Veterans. *Am J Psychiatry.* 154:1690–1695.

5

Post-Traumatic Stress Disorder and Chronic Pain

Jennifer Jane Runnals, Ph.D., Elizabeth Van Voorhees, Ph.D., and Patrick S. Calhoun, Ph.D.

Post-traumatic stress disorder (PTSD) and chronic pain result in human suffering (Geisser et al. 1996) and lead to economic burden due to lost productivity (Jenewein et al. 2009) and increased healthcare utilization (Von Korff et al. 1990; Schnurr et al. 2000). In the last two decades researchers have begun to focus on the simultaneous presentation of these conditions. The prevalence of comorbidity and the particularly intractable nature of these conditions when co-occurring has been well documented (Hickling and Blanchard 1992; Otis et al. 2006), and explanatory models have been proposed to account for high rates of co-occurrence. Recent studies have begun to provide evidence that will assist in refinement of these explanatory models, leading to better detection and treatment and reduced chronicity and severity for those diagnosed with comorbid PTSD and chronic pain.

This chapter reviews the literature on the co-occurrence of PTSD and chronic pain; including prevalence rates, predictors of the development of comorbid chronic pain and PTSD, models explicating etiological and maintaining factors accounting for comorbidity, assessment, and treatment approaches for comorbid presentations of PTSD and chronic pain. The chapter concludes with suggested directions for future research. This review does not include information regarding treatments that target PTSD or chronic pain separately (e.g., exposure treatments for PTSD or cognitive therapy for chronic pain), and readers are referred to reviews by Iverson, Lester, and Resick (2011) and Andrew (2009) for information about these treatments.

Much of the literature on comorbid chronic pain and PTSD lacks delineation of the temporal relationship between the two. For example, studies do not identify whether a chronic pain condition may be etiologically related to the trauma such as injury associated with a motor vehicle accident or non-etiological such as chronic lower back pain without a precipitating—or trauma-related injury. Published studies rarely document whether chronic pain was present prior to the traumatic event. Further, for research purposes, chronic pain is often limited to pain with known etiology (e.g., a disease or injury) that has lasted three or more months and thus may exclude pain-related conditions with no known etiology (i.e., pain without associated injury or disease process). In clinical practice, chronic pain may refer to these pain conditions with documented physical etiology, or to functional pain syndromes with no known, or poorly understood, etiology. In this review, the pain syndrome or pain site will be identified if done so in the literature and pertinent to the review.

PREVALENCE OF PTSD AND CHRONIC PAIN

Estimates of lifetime prevalence for PTSD have ranged from 6.4–9% in population studies conducted in the United States (Breslau et al. 2004; Kessler et al. 2005). In a review of national population surveys, the 12-month prevalence rate of PTSD ranged from 1.3% in Australia to 3.5% in the United States, with women, unmarried persons, and those with low income and less education having a greater risk for PTSD and other anxiety disorders (Baumeister and Harter 2007). Rates of chronic pain are greater than those for PTSD; studies of chronic pain prevalence across various countries have shown rates ranging from 10% to 23% (Blyth et al. 2001; Catala et al. 2002; Ng, Tsui, and Chan 2002) and, similar to PTSD, women report greater rates of chronic pain than men (Rustoen et al. 2004). The incidence of chronic pain in samples of persons injured in accidents (e.g., Jenewein et al. 2009) or in treatment-seeking samples is even greater, with rates reaching 44–50% (Elliot et al. 1999).

CO-OCCURRENCE OF PTSD AND CHRONIC PAIN

The co-occurrence of PTSD and chronic pain has been estimated at 7–8% lifetime prevalence in the general population (Von Korff et al. 2005). An international study of chronic neck and back pain showed that those reporting pain were three times more likely to have PTSD (Demyttenaere, Bruffaerts, and Lee 2007). In the United States, chronic musculoskeletal pain is associated with a fourfold increased risk for PTSD (Cox and McWilliams 2002). Shipherd et al. (2007) noted that 66% of veterans with PTSD carried a diagnosis of chronic pain, and symptoms of PTSD have shown a significant positive association with levels of pain severity (DeCarvalho 2010).

Given that patients with chronic pain and PTSD may be managed in various medical and mental health service settings, there has been interest in rates of PTSD among patients presenting for chronic pain treatment as well as rates of chronic pain among patients presenting for PTSD treatment. When compared to primary care patients with other anxiety disorders and patients with trauma exposure but no PTSD diagnosis, primary care patients with PTSD report two to three times greater likelihood of a number of physical ailments such as chronic lung disease and arthritis (Weisberg et al. 2002), even after controlling for health risk behaviors that are increased in patients with PTSD. Primary care patients with PTSD also exhibit a greater range and greater occurrence of pain-related health problems including back pain (Weisberg et al. 2002), fibromyalgia, and migraine headaches (Sareen et al. 2007). In a sample of 528 veterans in primary care, 40% reported moderate to severe pain, and more than half of these veterans reported significant symptoms of emotional distress (Sherbourne et al. 2009). Among patients in treatment for chronic pain, one-third to one-half of patients have been diagnosed with PTSD or report significant levels of PTSD symptomology (Geisser et al. 1996; Asmundson et al. 2009).

GENDER AND VETERAN STATUS

Women report higher prevalence rates of PTSD and of chronic pain as well as higher rates of exposure to interpersonal violence (Dutton et al. 2006). The published literature on rates of co-occurring chronic pain and PTSD in women primarily focuses on the experience of interpersonal violence (i.e., trauma that includes physical or sexual violence or threat of such by a women's partner (Saltzman et al 1999). In a recent study of 84 women with abuse histories, 77% reported chronic pain and 80% met criteria for PTSD based upon self-report of symptomology (Humphreys et al. 2010). Greater pain ratings were associated with higher levels of PTSD, higher levels of depression symptoms, and greater length of the abusive relationship. Studies of women veterans have reported rates of interpersonal violence in some samples as high as 74% (e.g. Campbell et al. 2008).

In contrast to women's greater exposure to interpersonal violence, men show greater rates of exposure to other types of trauma, including combat. Among 129 male U.S. Vietnam era combat-veterans with PTSD, 80% reported chronic pain (Beckham et al. 1997). Similarly, among Canadian veterans with PTSD, almost all participants reported clinically significant levels of pain (Poundja, Fikretoglu, and Brunet 2006). In a separate study, half of veterans enrolled in comprehensive treatment for chronic pain (primarily men with leg, back, and neck pain) met criteria for PTSD (Otis et al. 2010). Despite controlling for depression, these veterans with chronic pain and PTSD reported significantly greater pain-related affective distress compared to veterans with chronic pain alone. However, pain rating scores were similar between veterans with and without PTSD, indicating that, while pain intensity is comparable, veterans with PTSD are more distressed by their chronic pain. It is not clear whether this greater distress is associated with the etiology of the pain (e.g., whether the pain is trauma-related), reduced ability to cope with chronic pain, or both. Similar results have been found in women veterans, although they also report greater bodily pain ratings when chronic pain and PTSD co-occur (Asmundson et al. 2004).

In looking at 1,129 male and female veterans in primary care, Haskell et al. (2010) found that there were no differences in the rate of men (62%) and women (65%) reporting clinically significant pain on the day of appointment, though more men (33%) than women (21%) screened positive for PTSD. Other studies suggest chronic pain may be more frequently reported by women veterans diagnosed with PTSD (Kerns et al. 2003; Haskell et al. 2006). A recent study of male and female veterans who served in Iraq and Afghanistan showed chronic widespread pain (a more restrictive definition of chronic pain that requires chronic pain in four quadrants of the body) in 27% of men and 37% of women (Helmer et al. 2009). For veterans in whom a diagnosis of PTSD was more likely (i.e. they were positive on three of four screening questions for PTSD), 38% reported chronic pain—a total of 20% of this non-treatment-seeking population had co-occurring probable PTSD and chronic widespread pain. Other recent assessments of Operation Enduring Freedom/Operation Iraqi Freedom (OEF/OIF) veterans seeking care in the

Veterans Administration indicated that 47% were reporting at least mild pain and 28% moderate to severe pain (Gironda et al. 2006), that women veterans are experiencing greater post-deployment pain, and that both male and female veterans are experiencing increases in pain during the time since returning from Iraq or Afghanistan (Haskell et al. 2011).

PREDICTORS OF COMORBID PTSD AND CHRONIC PAIN

Although many traumas are not associated with injury, for those that are, two aspects of the injury and recovery from it are suggested to play a role in the development of chronic pain: injury severity and pain severity. While some researchers have noted a relationship between the severity of the traumatic injury and subsequent chronic pain conditions (e.g. Van Loey et al. 2003), these findings have primarily been reported among burn patients, a unique traumatic injury in which the treatment and recovery are known to elicit ongoing and significant pain. In contrast, others have found that the severity of post-trauma psychological distress is as integral to the development of chronic pain as injury severity (West et al. 2010) or that injury severity does not predict development of chronic pain (Jenewein et al. 2009).

Similarly, Patterson and colleagues (2006) found that acute injury-related pain was not a significant predictor of chronic pain, but was a better predictor of PTSD symptoms than length of hospital stay or the total body surface area damaged by burns. In two recent investigations, high levels of injury-related pain were a strong predictor of chronic pain (Liedl et al. 2010) and PTSD (Bryant et al. 2009). Importantly, pain has not been found to be significantly related to injury severity in some studies (Norman et al. 2007). This suggests that preexisting individual differences in pain-related cognitive and affective factors (e.g., pain perception differences, beliefs associated with pain, fearfulness of pain, etc.) are influential in the development of co-occurring PTSD and chronic pain, and that preexisting psychological factors influence the sensory experience of peritraumatic pain (Melzak and Katz 2004).

Unfortunately, in most published injury-related trauma studies it is not clear whether patients who report ongoing accident-related pain had preexisting chronic pain or past exposure to traumatic events or injuries.

This is important as a greater number of lifetime traumas may be associated with greater likelihood of ongoing medical conditions such as chronic pain (Sledjeski et al. 2008). It is also unclear from published studies whether other accident-related variables differ between those with and without chronic pain (Jenewein et al. 2009). For example, patient experience of pain during the traumatic event is often not assessed, which may be an important gap, given that peritraumatic pain (Glynn et al. 2007; Kuhn 2004) and affective distress associated with peritraumatic pain (Norman et al. 2007) have been identified as risk factors for PTSD.

As noted in a review by Beck and Clapp (2011), findings from prospective studies of the development of PTSD and chronic pain after injury (e.g., Sterling et al. 2003, 2005, 2006) indicate that early injury-related pain ratings predict the development of PTSD symptoms, which in turn predict the development of chronic pain. Early affective distress may either influence pain ratings or the ability to cope with pain, which affects the perception of pain. Thus, early injury-related pain ratings are likely confounded by trauma-related distress. Traumas resulting in more severe injury, and thus more pain, may also be more likely to result in PTSD, which then increases the risk of developing chronic pain. In other words, there could be a relationship between injury severity or peritraumatic pain and chronic pain that is affected by the development of PTSD. If PTSD potentiates the development of chronic pain, this might also explain why non-trauma-related pain conditions are common among patients with PTSD. There is some empirical support for a meditational model in which PTSD accounts for the relationship between violence-related trauma and pain-related symptoms (Campbell et al. 2008).

Clarifying the temporal relationship of chronic pain and PTSD is hampered by the limited number of longitudinal studies and the difficulty of conducting prospective longitudinal studies (i.e., it is difficult to obtain baseline data when there is limited ability to predict trauma exposure). In addition, many studies of comorbidity do not differentiate between cases of chronic pain that might be linked to the traumatic event versus cases where the pain-related condition is unrelated to the index trauma. Despite these impediments, there has been significant advancement toward understanding how these two conditions might potentiate or exacerbate each other. These theories are reviewed in the next section.

THEORIES EXPLAINING THE RELATIONSHIP BETWEEN PTSD AND CHRONIC PAIN

There is substantial evidence that poor physical health is an outcome of exposure to trauma, especially among persons who develop chronic PTSD (Schnurr and Green 2004). Similar to the relationship between trauma exposure, PTSD, and health, there is growing evidence that PTSD mediates the relationship between trauma exposure and chronic pain (Wuest et al. 2009, 2010) and that, for some persons, the relationship between PTSD and chronic pain may be mediated by depression (Poundja, Fikretoglu, and Brunet 2006; Roth et al. 2008).

For example, in a longitudinal study of 90 patients admitted to intensive care after an accident, PTSD symptoms 2 weeks post-injury predicted the presence or absence of chronic pain three years post-injury (Jenewein et al. 2009). All of the patients with PTSD (n = 12) reported chronic pain related to their injury, and those with chronic pain reported significantly greater disability, more days missed from work, and greater healthcare utilization. Turk and Okifuji (1996) found that, among patients with PTSD, even those without trauma-related physical injuries reported more pain than non-PTSD patients and were more likely to receive prescriptions for opiates and analgesics than non-PTSD patients.

A number of models or theories have been proposed to explain the relationship between PTSD and chronic pain. These theories tend to focus on aspects of the relationship between PTSD and chronic pain such as Sharp and Harvey's Mutual Maintenance Model (2001), which places emphasis on cognitive and behavioral factors common to both conditions. Others borrow from the neurobiological literature on the relationship between chronic stress and poor health (McEwen and Stellar 1993), conceptualizing PTSD as a specific and severe form of ongoing stress that results in failure to achieve homeostasis or allostasis. A number of these models are reviewed below.

PSYCHOLOGICAL MECHANISMS

The Mutual Maintenance Model, proposed by Sharp and Harvey (2001), is based on recognition of the significant overlap of physiological, affective, behavioral, and cognitive factors that separately were observed or hypothesized to maintain PTSD and chronic pain. Seven factors were implicated in maintaining both disorders: (1) attentional biases; (2) anxiety sensitivity (a tendency to respond to even harmless physical symptoms with fear); (3) persistent reminders of trauma; (4) avoidant coping style; (5) depression and reduced behavioral activation; (6) increased pain perception; and (7) increased demand on cognitive resources. These factors were presumed to interact and have a synergistic effect on these co-occurring conditions. For example, perception of pain may activate trauma memories, both of which heighten physiological arousal. This increased physiological activation would contribute to increased avoidance of activities that may increase pain, which decreases physical conditioning and raises the likelihood of more physical pain.

Subsequent to the introduction of Sharp and Harvey's model, Asmundson et al. (2002) proposed The Shared Vulnerability Model, which they conceptualized as an extension of the Mutual Maintenance Model (Asmundson and Katz 2009). The Shared Vulnerability Model places anxiety sensitivity in an etiological role, thus predisposing people for the development of both PTSD and chronic pain. Anxiety sensitivity is believed to add to emotional reactions experienced during trauma by virtue of the alarm related to increased physiological responses during activation of the autonomic nervous system. This Shared Vulnerability Model also recognizes that other preexisting psychological (e.g., greater sensitivity to feelings of lost control (Palyo and Beck 2005) and physiological vulnerabilities (e.g., genetic variations or lowered threshold for sympathetic nervous system activation) may place a person at greater risk for comorbid PTSD and chronic pain. Similarly, Otis et al. (2003) incorporate both predisposing biological and psychological vulnerability for PTSD and chronic pain in their adaptation of Barlow's Triple Vulnerability Model (Barlow 2000, 2002). In their model, Otis et al. proposed a genetic liability for the development of chronic pain and PTSD that is realized when the person is exposed to trauma in the context of accompanying psychological risk factors (e.g., perceived lack of control, poor coping skills, low social support, negative affect, and so on).

The Shared and Triple Vulnerability Models highlight the role of biological vulnerabilities and some biological changes in the onset and maintenance of both PTSD and chronic pain. Asmundson and Katz (2009) suggest that hyperarousal associated with autonomic nervous system activation is an adaptive response during acute stress, but that it becomes pathogenic when ongoing, as in both

PTSD and chronic pain. Injury in the context of trauma would similarly evoke neurobiological processes that are acutely adaptive, but that when chronically activated may heighten decrements in physical functioning and health. Thus, chronic anxiety-related physiological activation, whether precipitated by injury or not, may prompt repeated neural and hormonal changes. As these changes accumulate they contribute to poor health—including chronic pain. This view is supported by numerous studies showing a relationship between PTSD and poor health (Schnurr and Green 2004).

Asmundson and Katz (2009) and Beck and Clapp (2011) provide excellent reviews of studies including participants with PTSD and chronic pain that addressed the component parts of these models. There is evidence to support increased attentional biases related to both PTSD and pain syndromes in those with both conditions. In contrast, attentional biases have not been convincingly demonstrated in persons who have chronic pain but not PTSD (Asmundson and Katz 2009). There is evidence to support the relationship of anxiety sensitivity to both PTSD and chronic pain (Asmundson and Katz 2009), though establishing anxiety sensitivity as preceding the onset of either disorder is challenging.

Presently, no studies have explored how trauma reminders may or may not cue pain and vice versa, though one study has shown that increased levels of reexperiencing symptoms are associated with increased pain and disability (Beckham et al. 1997). A recent prospective longitudinal study of 824 hospitalized trauma patients provided evidence that the development of chronic pain symptoms is integrally tied to the development of hyperarousal and reexperiencing symptoms, and that this relationship is reciprocal (Liedl et al. 2010). Specifically, the relationship between PTSD reexperiencing and hyperarousal symptoms and pain symptoms became stronger over the period of assessment, and hyperarousal symptoms at the three-month assessment mediated the relationship between pain at the time of injury and chronic pain symptoms one year post-injury. In addition, continuing pain symptoms at three months predicted hyperarousal symptoms at the one year assessment. This study is a rare example of prospective work that allows for causal inferences, and provides strong support for the Mutual Maintenance Model. Two other factors highlighted in Sharp and Harvey's Mutual Maintenance Model, the role of increased avoidance and increases in cognitive demand (Beck and Clapp 2011), have not been examined empirically.

Contrary to the proposed increased pain perception of people with chronic pain and PTSD (Sharp and Harvey 2001), participants with PTSD have shown reduced pain perception in laboratory-based investigations (Geuze et al. 2007). Reduced perception of pain was associated with altered neural responses in the hippocampus, amygdala, and bilateral insular cortex. Follow-up studies of Dutch military veterans have shown that veterans with PTSD reported less pain than either non-combat veterans or non-veteran controls despite having similar warm and cold detection thresholds, the latter suggesting that differences in pain threshold are not attributable to sensory or attentional deficits (Kraus et al. 2009). In a study of women veterans, Strigo et al. (2010) noted a reduction in pain sensitivity in those with PTSD, but not in non-PTSD controls. Additionally, the authors noted that the patterns of neuronal activity suggest that women with PTSD were modulating emotions in such as way as to avoid the pain. It is not known whether the pain triggered reexperiencing symptoms, which then resulted in avoidance, or whether similar avoidance patterns would be present whether the pain is evocative of trauma or not. Given that these studies are cross-sectional it is not possible to determine with certainty whether differences in pain perception precede or follow onset of PTSD (Kraus et al. 2009).

One hypothesized explanation for reduced pain perception among those with PTSD has been stress-induced analgesia (Pitman et al. 1990; Foa et al. 1992). A study by Defrin et al. (2008) shed light on this counterintuitive finding of reduced pain perception by showing that, when compared to participants with other anxiety disorders, those with PTSD experienced hypoalgesia or hyperalgesia depending upon whether the stimuli were at or above the threshold for pain. Similar findings have been reported in comparisons of predictable pain (resulting in hypoanalgesia) to unpredictable pain resulting in hyperanalgesia (Ploghaus 2003).

It may be that factors unique to PTSD and not seen in other anxiety disorders, such as numbing and dissociative symptoms, affect how pain is perceived or processed, and that the extent to which the pain is predictable or alarming may affect whether the stimuli induces hypo- or hyperanalgesia. Asmundson and Katz (2009) suggest that a response of hypo- or hyperanalgesia could be influenced by whether the stimuli is perceived as *anxiety* provoking (e.g., unpredictable and oriented toward the future) versus *fear* provoking (e.g., immediate threat based) and that these distinctions may point to differences in how these stimuli are processed. Laboratory studies have shown that stimuli that invoke fear are responded to with less pain than non-fearful stimuli (Rhudy et al. 2004). Dissociation or psychological numbing symptoms may provide the mechanism by which sensitivity to pain is at times reduced in patients with PTSD, which could occur with greater pain stimuli, less predictable pain stimuli, and pain stimuli that produce fear as opposed to anxiety. Whether pain perception or intensity differs according to whether or not the person's trauma memory network includes a sensory pain component is not known (Lang 1979; Foa and Kozak 1986).

Different patterns of cardiovascular and neuronal activity are seen in participants with PTSD who report dissociative symptoms during exposure to trauma cues compared to PTSD participants who do not dissociate. For example, during dissociation, participants with PTSD do not exhibit the increases in venous return conductance (GVR), heart rate, or blood pressure seen in PTSD participants who do not dissociate (Lanius et al. 2006). In women with PTSD, reduced pain perception is associated with decreased activation of areas of the brain that correspond with avoidance (which is associated with numbing), including the right anterior *insula* (Strigo et al. 2010). Recently Ludascher et al. (2010) demonstrated that pain sensitivity is lower during dissociated states among participants with a personality disorder that is closely associated with extensive history of trauma exposure. In addition, Asmundson and Katz point to research on dysregulation of the endogenous opiod system in those with PTSD or chronic pain. This dysregulation (increased release of endogenous opiods), which has been linked to an increase in numbing symptoms of PTSD, may be an adaptation to chronic fear and pain.

More recently, Martin et al. (2010) examined an adaptation of Turk's Diathesis-Stress Model of chronic pain and disability. Turk included trauma exposure as one precipitating factor in his model of the development of chronic pain and disability; Martin et al. adapted this model to more specifically indicate the presence of PTSD (not just trauma exposure) in the pathogenesis of chronic pain. This adaptation of Turk's model suggests that anxiety sensitivity and pain intensity directly affect fear of pain, that fear of pain and perceived pain intensity directly affect symptoms of PTSD, and that PTSD symptoms and ongoing pain intensity have a direct effect on chronic pain and disability.

The Mutual Maintenance, Shared Vulnerability, Triple Vulnerability, and Diathesis-Stress models have proposed factors and organizational structures that have roles in the etiology and/or maintenance of co-occurring PTSD and chronic pain. While models of chronic pain invoking cognitive and physiological variables illuminate the relationship between psychological factors, behavior, and amplification or perception of pain, they do not address biological mechanisms that may causally link PTSD and chronic pain. Though far from being fully understood, some current attempts to explain underlying mechanisms are reviewed below.

BIOLOGICAL MECHANISMS

Within a biopsychosocial framework, PTSD and functional pain syndromes have both been conceptualized as resulting from an overactivated stress response system that may have been compromised prior to the index trauma. For example, McLean et al. (2005) propose that neurobiological mechanisms operating within central stress systems may account for both the development of chronic pain conditions and for the development of PTSD. However, they also postulate that these neurobiological changes are influenced or affected by cognitive-behavioral factors. This view of the development of PTSD and chronic pain may be supported by prospective studies showing that, in participants injured at the time of trauma, symptoms of both disorders develop and remit in a parallel process (Beck and Clapp 2011), and that the relationship between PTSD and pain symptoms strengthens over time (Liedl et al. 2010). Further, McClean points to animal studies as further evidence for a causal relationship between stress (i.e., trauma exposure and non-recovery) and subsequent changes in neural circuitry associated with sensory experience of pain (i.e., nociception).

It is beyond the scope of this chapter to review the entire network of neurobiological systems implicated in the relationship between chronic pain and PTSD. However, one neuroendocrine circuit, the hypothalamic-pituitary-adrenal (HPA) axis, discussed elsewhere in this book, has been studied in relation to both PTSD and chronic pain disorders. This system interacts in complex ways with other bodily systems to regulate responses to pain and stress. As an introduction to the neurobiological substrates of the link between PTSD and chronic pain, we briefly discuss research on the potential involvement of the HPA axis and related systems in PTSD and chronic pain.

Chronic pain disorders are highly comorbid with both PTSD and depression, and the expression of symptoms across and among disorders can be affected by complex interactions of each of the hormones of the HPA axis with multiple bodily systems. For example, though major depression and PTSD have different profiles in terms of cortisol secretion, both are associated with hypersecretion of corticotrophin-releasing hormone. During acute stress corticotrophin-releasing hormone is associated with analgesia, but there is evidence that chronic exposure to stress may result in hyperalgesia, precisely the opposite effect (Lariviere and Melzack 2000). As such, PTSD, depression, and some chronic pain-related disorders such as irritable bowel syndrome may be linked by chronic overproduction of corticotrophin-releasing hormone (Chrousos 1998; Heim 2000). In contrast to the corticotrophin-releasing hormone hypersecretion association with PTSD, chronic fatigue syndrome and fibromyalgia have been associated with decreased corticotrophin-releasing hormone secretion (Crofford et al. 1996; Chruosus 1998; Tanriverdi et al. 2007). However, all of these disorders are characterized by enhanced negative feedback suppression of the HPA axis by cortisol (Crofford, Engleberg, and Demitrack 1996; Heim et al. 2000; Ehlert et al. 2001; McBeth et al. 2005, 2007; Yehuda 2006; Tanriverdi et al. 2007; Galli et al. 2009).

Dysregulated cortisol secretion may interact with many other systems to produce symptomatology. For example, Vierck (2006) proposed a mechanism by which the stress of acute injury can lead to the chronic widespread pain of fibromyalgia. Specifically, after acute injury, sympathetic activation leads to vasoconstriction in peripheral tissues and thus to ischemia and inflammation. In cases of inadequate healing, peripheral sensory receptors become sensitized due to chronic activation, and chronic nociceptive input ultimately results in the central sensitization of pain processes through upregulation of N-methyl D-aspartate (NMDA) receptors. Increasing pain sensitivity, in turn, activates the HPA axis and sympathetic system, creating a vicious cycle (Vierck 2006).

Finally, cortisol has been found to inhibit immune function. There are numerous studies suggesting a relationship between chronic stress, increased cortisol secretion, and alterations in immune functioning. In contrast, increased adaptive coping may enhance immune functioning (Kiecolt-Glaser et al. 2002). If psychological distress, such as severe stress and ongoing pain, impedes healing via suppressed immune functioning, it seems plausible that this delay in recovery would facilitate the transformation of acute injury and pain conditions to chronic conditions. For example, as proposed by Vierck (2006) with respect to fibromyalgia, extended healing and thus increased exposure to pain could result in changes in nociception. Diminished inhibition of immune function associated with hypocortisolism has been found in autoimmune and inflammatory diseases such as rheumatoid arthritis (Chrousos 1995; O'Toole and Catts 2008). In summary, there are multiple mechanisms by which severe or chronic stress can alter the functioning of the HPA axis. Evidence for HPA axis dysregulation in PTSD has pointed to increased corticotrophin-releasing hormone, increased negative feedback inhibition of the HPA axis by cortisol, and dysregulation of cortisol secretion. Each of these disruptions can interact with multiple bodily systems including immune/inflammatory systems and peripheral and central pain processing systems to create disruptions leading to chronic pain syndromes.

Overall these psychological and biological models explicate how myriad variables across behavioral, cognitive, affective, and physiological domains may play a role in the onset and maintenance of PTSD and chronic pain. While the role of neurobiological mechanisms may be implicit in these models, it would be useful to more explicitly incorporate neurobiological mechanisms into the existing frameworks. Such a synthesis would highlight the suspected under-lying neurobiological processes that are influenced by distress and that contribute to further changes and decrements in health and chronic pain.

Such a Psycho-Neurobiological Model of Pain and PTSD (PMPP) can be seen in Figure 5.1. Under the broad headings of physical, psychological, and environmental factors, are examples of concepts implicated or having demonstrated support for influencing PTSD and chronic pain (e.g., that anxiety sensitivity is an underlying factor common to the development of both PTSD and chronic pain). These broad factors are inclusive of cognitive, behavioral, affective, physiological, neuroendocrine, genetic, and social domains. The model also emphasizes the interrelationships of the factors and invokes a developmental approach to the onset and maintenance of comorbid PTSD and chronic pain. This representation builds upon prior models (Sharp and Harvey 2001; Otis et al. 2003; Gatchel 2004; Asmundson and Katz 2009), but expands upon those models to capture the role of neurobiological changes (acute and chronic) as well as the implicated time

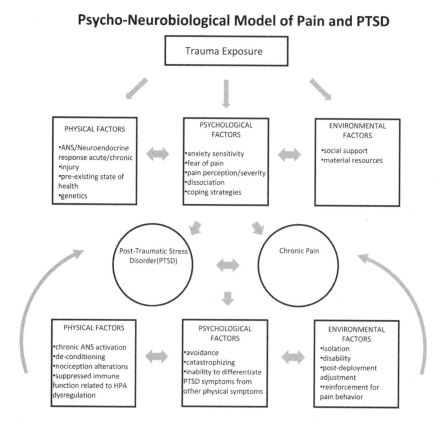

Psycho-Neurobiological Model of Pain and PTSD

Figure 5.1.

course and worsening of psychological and physical symptoms over time. Such neurobiological changes, as well as changes across the other factors, may provide an explanation for the chronicity and intractability of these conditions.

For example, though Vierck (2006) does not specifically consider the role of ongoing psychological stress in his model, he does emphasize the role of stress system activation in his hypothesis that peripheral injury can lead to central sensitization of pain processes observed in fibromyalgia, which is consistent with approaches by other stress and pain researchers (Gatchel 2004). From the perspective of this Psycho-Neurobiological Model, Vierck's work suggests the possibility of examining how trauma-related amplification of stress system activation across physical, psychological, and environmental factors may initiate and exacerbate the development of chronic pain syndromes.

Importantly, the model also draws attention to, but leaves undefined, an understudied aspect of comorbid chronic pain and PTSD, which is how the relationship between pain and PTSD unfolds, and more specifically whether the relationship between PTSD and pain unfolds differently when pain is not etiological to trauma. Further research is needed to determine the utility of the model and to test aspects of the relationships. For example, if stress-related changes in HPA axis functioning are present in comorbid presentations of PTSD and chronic pain, one hypothesis is that normal HPA axis functioning could be restored by successful treatment. However, some level of chronic pain might still be experienced (e.g., due to changes in nociception), even if the person shows successful adaptation to self-management of pain. This model provides a framework for the generation and organization of new research and findings.

ASSESSMENT OF CO-OCCURRING PTSD AND CHRONIC PAIN

It is evident from the section on psychological and biological theories of co-occurring PTSD and chronic pain that numerous factors are implicated in the comorbid presentation of these disorders. The presence of physiological, affective, behavioral, and cognitive components and their discrete components such as attentional biases, anxiety sensitivity, reexperiencing and hyperarousal symptoms, avoidant coping style, depression, and increased pain perception, suggest that patient assessment will necessarily be multifactorial and influenced by theory, purpose of assessment, and other concerns. A number of broad and specific content areas are important when assessing the effect of chronic pain on psychological functioning. Otis (2007) provides an example of content areas to assess in a clinical pain interview that includes general clinical information such as psychosocial history, substance use, and affective status as well as specific information such as pain location, details of injury and/or onset of pain, pain rating, prior treatments and their effectiveness, pain triggers and reducers, and pain-related coping strategies.

Patients who undergo psychological treatment for chronic pain may or may not receive a mental health diagnosis related to pain, and that has not been a requirement in treatment studies (e.g., Otis et al. 2009). In addition to other prerequisites, to receive a mental health diagnosis of Pain Disorder using criteria from the fourth edition of the Diagnostic and Statistical Manual of

Mental Disorders (DSM-IV), the patient must have pain that causes clinically significant distress or impairment of functioning, and psychological factors need to play a role in the onset and/or maintenance of the pain. Presence of distress and impairment provide reasonable guidelines for determining whether a patient with chronic pain needs or would benefit from a psychological approach to pain management. As Turk and Okifuji (2002) noted, treatment for chronic pain may be unnecessary for adaptive copers, effective for patients for whom pain is affecting daily functioning, and in need of adaptation for those who are poorly functioning and interpersonally distressed. Determining level of functional impairment and the role of psychological factors may rely on clinical judgment, or clinicians may find it useful to administer standardized measures to assist in this decision. Numerous objective self-report measures have been developed that tap into various aspects of the experience of chronic pain such as pain intensity, physical functioning, the beliefs associated with pain, and affective distress accompanying chronic pain. These measures, which are reviewed below, are well-validated and have demonstrated utility for clinical care and research.

PAIN INTENSITY

Pain intensity is defined as how much hurt the person is feeling (Jensen and Karoly 2001). Three methods are available for measuring pain intensity: visual analogue scales, numerical rating scales, and verbal rating scales. As Jensen and Karoly (2001) note, patients are not as receptive to the visual analogue scales as the other options, in part due to their abstract quality. Dworkin et al. (2005) make specific recommendations on preferred numerical rating scales for inclusion in studies assessing chronic pain treatments (i.e., an 11 point scale ranging from 0 or 'no pain' to 10 or 'pain as bad as you can imagine') that is similarly useful in clinical settings. Pain intensity ratings are useful for both initial assessment and assessing progress; however, they are influenced by factors such as time of day, presence of others when ratings are made, and stress. These ratings have the greatest utility when they are averaged across a number of assessment conditions. Daily charting of pain ratings may be useful in identifying fluctuations in pain of which distressed chronic patients are often unaware.

PAIN QUALITY

The sensory and affective components of pain are distinct from level of pain and may be affected differently by varying pain-related treatments (Jensen 2003). One recommended tool is the Short-Form McGill Pain Questionnaire (SF-MPQ; Melzack 1987). This measure assesses the distress and unpleasantness associated with pain (Dworkin et al. 2005). Use of a touch-screen version of this form, even among computer novices, suggests it is equivalent in terms of validity and reliability to pencil and paper versions (Cook et al. 2004). As with the level of pain, recurrent pain quality assessment may be useful for capturing the treatment associated with changes in distress.

PHYSICAL FUNCTIONING

Two brief and broadly applicable measures are available for the assessment of disruption of physical functioning: the West Haven-Yale Multidimensional Pain Inventory (MPI; Kerns et al. 1985) and the Brief Pain Inventory (BPI; Cleeland and Ryan 1994). The 9 item Interference Scale of the MPI or the 7 item Pain Interference Scale of the BPI both yield scores assessing the disruption of pain in aspects of daily living (e.g., work, relationships with others, and enjoyment of activities). Dworkin et al. (2005) cautions that sleep disruption is not assessed in the MPI, which may necessitate use of additional measures. However, the full version of the MPI includes information that may be particularly useful in clinical settings such as the responses to pain behavior the patient receives from their significant other and the level of avoidance or engagement in a range of activities (household chores, outdoor work, activities away from home, social activities, and general activity). Both measures have demonstrated excellent psychometric properties (Keller et al. 2004) and are recommended by pain researchers from the Initiative on Methods, Measurement, and Pain Assessment in Clinical Trials or IMMPACT (2003).

PAIN BELIEFS AND THOUGHTS

Pain-related beliefs influence adjustment to chronic pain. Two measures that are useful in assessing beliefs are the Pain Beliefs and Perceptions Inventory (PBPI; Williams and Thorn 1989) and the Survey of Pain Attitudes-Revised (SOPA-R: Jensen, Turner, and Romano 2000). The PBPI includes several scales; higher scores on the Pain as Mystery scale are related to greater distress (Thorn 2004). In addition, the Self-Blame score may be particularly relevant in a patient with PTSD as self-blame is often a cognitive distortion present in patients with PTSD that is targeted during trauma treatment (Resick, Monson, and Chard 2007). The SOPA-R includes a Control scale that assesses perception of control over pain. Higher scores are linked to better adjustment to chronic pain (Jensen et al. 1994). The tendency to catastrophize or exaggerate threat is common in both PTSD and in poor adaptation to chronic pain. The Pain Catastrophizing Scale (PCS; Sullivan et al. 1995; Osman et al. 2000) assesses pain-related rumination, helplessness, and the tendency to exaggerate the worse possible outcome, and may inform the emphasis a clinician places on cognitive interventions for pain and PTSD.

READINESS FOR TREATMENT

Not all patients are ready for or benefit from self-management or psychological approaches to treating chronic pain. This readiness can be assessed via the Pain Stages of Change Questionnaire (Kerns et al. 1997). More recent and concise adaptations of this measure found in the Multidimensional Pain Readiness to Change Questionnaire (Nielson et al. 2003) and the Multidimensional Pain Readiness to Change Questionnaire Version 2 (Nielson et al. 2009) are available. For patients whose scores suggest they are not yet ready for self-management approaches, treatment may be prefaced by information and strategies that enhance readiness for change (e.g., psychoeducation regarding a biopsychosocial conceptualization of chronic pain, evaluation of current behavior, and homework charting pain ratings and their relationship to stress).

Overall these assessment tools may supplement clinicians' interviews as well as provide indications of progress during treatment. Approaches to treating comorbid PTSD and chronic pain are reviewed below.

INTEGRATED PSYCHOLOGICAL TREATMENTS FOR CO-OCCURRING PTSD AND CHRONIC PAIN

Integrated treatments for PTSD and chronic pain are in development. Until recently, psychological treatments for simultaneous presentations of these conditions were either not undertaken or treatments were presented sequentially, which significantly increases time in therapy. Research-informed suggestions for treatment and an integrated treatment with early indications of effectiveness are reviewed below.

COGNITIVE-BEHAVIORAL TREATMENTS

While evidence-based treatments for PTSD have as their goal the amelioration of trauma symptoms, psychological approaches to treating chronic pain focus on increasing adaptive responses that includes accepting the chronicity of pain, increasing effective coping, reducing suffering (Thorn 2004), reducing helplessness, increasing personal responsibility, and decreasing disability (Otis 2007). The manner in which these tasks are accomplished includes interventions such as cognitive restructuring (to alter maladaptive thoughts that exacerbate pain), relaxation training (to reduce physical tension that exacerbates pain), and activity pacing (to appropriately manage activity levels to prevent cyclical deconditioning and avoidance).

Given that those with PTSD and greater pain severity are not as responsive to treatment as PTSD patients with less severe pain (Taylor et al. 2001), and that some pain treatments are less effective in those with PTSD (Dunn et al. 2009), there has been interest in combining or integrating treatments for these disorders. For example, Shipherd (2006) published a case study outlining a Cognitive-Behavioral Therapy based trauma treatment for a survivor of a motor vehicle collision with PTSD and chronic pain. Shipherd (2006) incorporated exposure to benign but feared physiological sensations (interoceptive exposure) as a way of directly addressing the patient's elevated anxiety sensitivity.

Similarly, Wald et al. (2010) present preliminary data on five participants who completed an exposure-based trauma treatment that was preceded by interoceptive exposure. Interoceptive exposure appeared to reduce anxiety sensitivity, which was associated with reductions in pain. Shipherd (2006) suggested that other aspects of the trauma-focused Cognitive-Behavioral Therapy treatment (e.g., reduced avoidance consequent to exposure, cognitive restructuring) could be tailored to address both trauma and chronic pain content. It is not known whether the necessity of including behavioral components may differ depending upon, for example, whether the pain and trauma share the same etiology or how long-standing the chronic pain is.

In an earlier case series Shipherd et al. (2003) demonstrated that six women with treatment-resistant chronic pain resulting from a motor vehicle accident saw improvements in pain-related measures (e.g., reduced disability, reduced days spent in bed, return to employment), but not pain ratings, after completion of treatment for PTSD. Together the results of the case studies suggest that, in patients with trauma-related pain, treatments for PTSD that also target anxiety sensitivity (i.e., interoceptive exposure) effectively reduce PTSD symptoms and some aspects of pain-related symptoms. However, significant improvements in psychological symptoms associated with pain have not yet been achieved. Although studies with larger sample sizes are needed, results from these preliminary studies suggest that remission of both trauma and pain-related symptoms may require a treatment approach that integrates the active components of Cognitive-Behavioral Therapy interventions for both conditions.

There are early indications that an integrated psychotherapeutic PTSD-chronic pain treatment is effective in reducing both trauma and pain-related symptoms (Otis et al. 2009). Otis and colleagues report on development of a 12-session treatment that integrated aspects of Cognitive Processing Therapy and Cognitive-Behavioral Therapy treatment for chronic pain. Integration of the treatments was born out of empirical and anecdotal observations that each condition appeared to hinder remission of the other when being treated either separately or sequentially (Otis et al. 2009). The formation of the treatment was guided by clinical observations, consultation with fellow subject-matter experts, and knowledge of efficacious treatments for both conditions. Though this small pilot study of U.S. military veterans suffered significant attrition, the veterans who remained enrolled in the study experienced significant decreases in pain symptoms and no longer met criteria for PTSD. A randomized controlled trial to thoroughly investigate treatment efficacy recently concluded, and results are pending.

As integrated treatments for PTSD and chronic pain are nascent, there is little information regarding for whom they are necessary or successful. For example, integrated treatments could be most beneficial for those whose pain has a trauma etiology. On the other hand, co-occurring or sequential treatment may be sufficient in cases of comorbidity lacking a common etiology.

PREVENTION

There do not appear to be studies examining psychological approaches for prevention of co-occurring PTSD and chronic pain in the peritraumatic phase. However, there are intriguing and provocative results from a small number of studies examining the effect of morphine administration during the acute phase of physical trauma. For example, in an observational study of patients hospitalized after injuries, Bryant et al. (2009) found that acute administration of morphine was associated with reduced symptoms of PTSD. They speculate, based on animal models, that administration of opiates affected levels of norepinephrine, which then disrupted fear conditioning and consolidation of trauma memories. However, the authors also point out that administration of morphine may have lessened acute pain, which then resulted in fewer symptoms of PTSD. One could speculate that the trauma memory network (Foa and Kozak 1986) of patients whose pain is well-controlled either lacks a pain-related sensory component, or the pain-related memories are attenuated. These results replicate those found in children with burn injuries (Saxe et al. 2001). Saxe et al. (2001) speculate that peritraumatic administration of opiates could play a role in preventing PTSD, noting of course, that controlled trials are needed to examine this possibility. Unfortunately, neither acute nor chronic pain was reported in their investigation, thus it is unclear how peritraumatic administration of opiates may affect onset of chronic pain.

FUTURE RESEARCH

Despite advances in this area, many aspects of the relationship between PTSD and chronic pain have not been fully clarified. Further research is needed, and some of the potential advancement is likely to be derived from increasing specificity in the questions asked and carefully selecting study populations. For example, prospective studies of individuals who develop PTSD subsequent to an injury-related trauma may reveal relationships among variables that do not hold for patients with PTSD who develop unrelated chronic pain. The rates of co-occurring PTSD and chronic pain may also differ for these two populations. As Asmundson and Katz (2009) note, most of what is known about the relationship between chronic pain and PTSD is derived from studies of chronic musculoskeletal pain. Research with other pain populations and more clear delineation of the time course of pain and trauma are needed.

Asmundson and Katz (2009) also pointed to the need for longitudinal studies to better illuminate the influence of preexisting traits and vulnerabilities, such as anxiety sensitivity, in the onset and maintenance of PTSD and chronic pain. In addition to clearer understanding of these psychological variables, the field would benefit from inclusion of suspected neurobiological variables, which may contribute to understanding of the physical deconditioning and to the broader aspects of poor health that are seen in patients with PTSD and chronic pain.

Exciting developments are occurring in integrated psychological treatment for PTSD and chronic pain. As these treatments are tested, further questions will likely arise as to whether integrated treatments are necessary or beneficial, as well as if patients who may only need one treatment are better served by sequential rather than simultaneous treatment. Additionally, questions may surface regarding how newly integrated treatments can be adapted for even more specific populations, such as veterans with comorbid PTSD, chronic pain, and traumatic brain injury, or adapted for other technologies such as telemedicine. These treatment efficacy questions suggest that assessment of patients and awareness of the heterogeneity of pain and PTSD patients may be integral to matching patients to the least time-consuming and most efficacious services.

SUMMARY AND CONCLUSIONS

Patients with comorbid PTSD and chronic pain are more distressed and impaired than patients experiencing only one of these conditions (Geisser et al. 1996; Amir et al. 1997). Comorbid patients also are more refractory to treatment than patients with only one condition (Hickling and Blanchard 1992; Otis et al. 2006). While much is still unknown about the comorbidity of these conditions, we are in a better position today to detect patients who need assistance with these dual diagnoses and to provide beneficial psychological treatments. Though treating these comorbid conditions is of long-standing need and importance, it is particularly salient in the new and growing population of veterans of recent and ongoing conflicts. The hope is that they, as well as civilians who experience these difficulties, might experience better post-trauma adjustment, less disability, and optimal quality of life.

REFERENCES

American Psychiatric Association. 2000. *Diagnostic and Statistical Manual of Mental Disorders.* (4th Ed. ed.). Washington, DC: American Psychiatric Association.

Amir M, Kaplan Z, Neumann L, et al. 1997. Posttraumatic stress disorder, tenderness and fibromyalgia. *Journal of Psychosomatic Research.* 42:607–613.

Andrew L. 2009. Psychosocial interventions in the treatment of pain. In: Mehta N, Maloney G, Dhirendra B et al., editors. *Head, face, and neck pain science, evaluation and management: An interdisciplinary approach.* Hoboken, NJ: Wiley-Blackwell, pp 24–33.

Arguelles LM, Afari N, Buchwald DS, et al. 2006. A twin study of posttraumatic stress disorder symptoms and chronic widespread pain. *Pain.* 124:150–157.

Asmundson GJG, Coons MJ, Taylor S, et al. 2002. PTSD and the experience of pain: Research and clinical implications of shared vulnerability and mutual maintenance models. *Canadian Journal of Psychiatry.* 47:930–937.

Asmundson GJG, Katz J. 2009. Understanding the co-occurrence of anxiety disorders and chronic pain: state-of-the-art. *Depression and Anxiety.* 26:888–901.

Asmundson GJ, Wright KD, Stein MB 2004. Pain and PTSD symptoms in female veterans. *European Journal of Pain.* 8:345–350.

Asmundson GJ, Taylor S. 1996. Role of anxiety sensitivity in pain-related fear and avoidance. *Journal of Behavior Medicine.* 19:577–586.

Barlow DH. 2000. Unraveling the mysteries of anxiety and its disorders from the perspective of emotion theory. *American Psychologist.* 55:1247–1263.

Barlow DH. 2002. *Anxiety and Its Disorders*, 2nd ed. New York: Guilford Press.

Baumeister H, Harter M. 2007. Prevalence of mental disorders based on general population surveys. *Soci Psychiatry Psychiatr Epidemiology.* 42:537–546.

Beck JG, Clapp JD. 2011. A different kind of comorbidity: Understanding Posttraumatic Stress Disorder and chronic pain. *Psychological Trauma: Theory, Research, Practice, and Policy.* 1–8.

Beckham JC, Crawford AL, Feldman ME, et al. 1997. Chronic posttraumatic stress disorder and chronic pain in Vietnam combat veterans. *Journal of Psychosomatic Research.* 43(4):379–389.

Blyth FM, March LM, Brnabic AJ, et al. 2001. Chronic pain in Australia: A prevalence study. *Pain.* 89:127–134.

Breslau N, Lansing MI, Peterson EL, et al. 2004. Estimating PTSD in the community: Lifetime perspective and the impact of typical trauma events. *Psychological Medicine.* 34(5):889–898.

Bryant RA, Creamer M, O'Donnell M, et al. 2009. A study of the protective function of acute morphine administration on subsequent posttraumatic stress disorder. *Biological Psychiatry.* 65:438–440.

Campbell R, Greeson MR, Bybee D, et al. 2008. The co-occurrence of childhood sexual abuse, adult sexual assault, intimate partner violence, and sexual harassment: A meditational model of posttraumatic stress disorder and physical health outcomes. *Journal of Consulting and Clinical Psychology.* 76(2):194–207.

Catala E, Reig E, Artes M, et al. 2002. Prevalence of pain in the Spanish population: Telephone survey in 5000 homes. *European Journal of Pain.* 6(2):133–140.

Chrousos GP. 1998. Stressors, stress, and neuroendocrine integration of the adaptive response. The 1997 Hans Selye Memorial Lecture. *Ann N Y Acad Sci.* 851:311–335.

Cleeland CS, Ryan KM 1994. Pain assessment: Global use of the Brief Pain Inventory. *Ann Acad Med Singapore.* 23(2):129–138.

Cook AJ, Roberts DA, Henderson MD, et al. 2004. Electronic pain questionnaires: A randomized, crossover comparison with paper questionnaires for chronic pain assessment. *Pain.* 110:310–317.

Cox BJ, McWilliams LA. 2002. Mood and anxiety disorders in relation to chronic pain: evidence from the National Comorbidity Study. *Pain Research Management.* 5(suppl. A):11A.

Crofford LJ, Engleberg NC, Demitrack MA. 1996. Neurohormonal perturbations in fibromyalgia. *Baillieres Clin Rheumatol.* 10(2):365–378. (DOI: S0950 3579(96)80022-7 [pii]).

DeCarvalho LT. 2010. Important missing links in the treatment of chronic low back pain patients. *Journal of Musculoskeletal Pain.* 18(1):11–22.

Defrin R, Ginzburg K, Solomon Z, et al. 2008. Quantitative testing of pain perception in subjects with PTSD—implications for the mechanism of co-existence between PTSD and chronic pain. *Pain.* 138:450–459.

Demyttenaere K, Bruffaerts R, Lee S. 2007. Mental disorders among persons with chronic back or neck pain: results from the World Mental Health Surveys. *Pain.* 129:332–342.

Dunn AS, Passmore SR, Burke J, et al. 2009. A cross-sectional analysis of clinical outcomes following chiropractic care in veterans with and without posttraumatic stress disorder. *Military Medicine.* 174(6):578–583.

Dutton MA, Green BL, Kaltman SI, et al. 2006. Intimate partner violence, PTSD, and adverse health outcomes. *Journal of Interpersonal Violence.* 21:955–968.

Dworkin R, Turk DC, Farrar JR, et al. 2005. Core outcome measures for chronic pain trials: IMMPACT recommendations. *Pain.* 113(1–2):9–19.

Elliot AM, Smith BH, Penny KI, et al. 1999. The epidemiology of chronic pain in the community. *Lancet.* 354:1248–1252.

Ehlert U, Gaab J, Heinrichs M. 2001. Psychoneuroendocrinological contributions to the etiology of depression, posttraumatic stress disorder, and stress-related bodily disorders: the role of the hypothalamus-pituitary-adrenal axis. *Biological Psychiatry.* 57:141–152.

Foa EB, Kozak MJ. 1986. Emotional processing of fear: Exposure to corrective information. *Psychological Bulletin.* 99:20–35.

Foa EB, Zinbarg R, Rothbaum BO. 1992. Uncontrollability and unpredictability in post-traumatic stress disorder: an animal model. *Psychological Bulletin* 112:218–238.

Galli U, Gaab J, Ettlin DA, et al. 2009. Enhance negative feedback sensitivity of the hypothalamus-pituitary-adrenal axis in chronic myogenous facial pain. *Eur J Pain.* 13(6):600–605. (DOI: S1090-3801(08)00170-5 [pii]).

Gatchel R. 2004. Comorbidity of chronic pain and mental health disorders: The biopsychosocial perspective. *American Psychologist.* 795–805.

Geisser ME, Roght RS, Bachman JE, et al. 1996. The relationship between symptoms of post-traumatic stress disorder and pain, affective disturbance and disability among patients with accident and non-accident related pain. *Pain.* 66:207–214.

Gironda RJ, Clark ME, Massengale JP, et al. 2008. Pain among veterans of Operations Enduring Freedom and Iraqi Freedom. *Pain Medicine.* 7(4):339–343.

Glynn SM, Shetty V, Elliot-Brown K, et al. 2007. Chronic posttraumatic stress disorder after facial injury: a 1-year prospective cohort study. *Journal of Trauma.* 62:410–418.

Geuze E, Westenberg HGM, Jochims A, et al. 2007. Altered pain processing in veterans with posttraumatic stress disorder. *Archives of General Psychiatry.* 64:76–85.

Haskell S, Ning Y, Krebs E, et al. 2012. Prevalence of painful musculoskeletal pain conditions in female and male Veterans in seven years after returning from deployment in Operation Iraqi Freedom. *Clinical Journal of Pain.* 28:163–167.

Haskell SG, Heapy A, Reid MC, et al. 2006. The prevalence and age-related characteristics in a sample of women veterans receiving primary care. *Journal of Women's Health.* 15:862–869.

Haskell SG, Gordon KS, Mattocks K, et al. 2010. Gender differences in rates of depression, PTSD, pain, obesity, and military sexual trauma among Connecticut was veterans of Iraq and Afghanistan. *Journal of Women's Health.* 19(2):267–271.

Heim C, Ehlert U, Hellhammer, DH. 2000. The potential role of hypocortisolism in the pathophysiology of stress-related bodily disorders. *Psychoneuroendocrinology.* 25(1):1–35. (DOI: S0306-4530(99)00035-9 [pii]).

Helmer DA, Chandler HK, Quigley KS, et al. 2009. Chronic widespread pain, mental health, and physical role function in OEF/OIF veterans. *Pain Medicine.* 10(7):1174–1182.

Hickling EJ, Blanchard EB. 1992. Post-traumatic stress disorder and motor vehicle accidents. *Journal of Anxiety Disorders.* 6:285–291.

Humphreys J, Cooper, BA, Miaskowski C. 2010. Differences in depression, posttraumatic stress disorder, and lifetime trauma exposure in formerly abused women with mild versus moderate to severe chronic pain. *Journal of Interpersonal Violence.* 25(12):2316–2338.

Initiative on Methods, Measurement, and Pain Assessment in Clinical Trials (IMMPACT). 2011. Available at: http://www.immpact.org/. Accessed Jan 31, 2012.

Iverson K, Lester K, Resick P. 2011. Psychosocial Treatments. In: Benedek D, Wynn G, editors. *Clinical Manual for the Management of Posttraumatic Stress Disorder.* Arlington, VA: American Psychiatric Publishing, Inc. 157–203.

Jenewein J, Wittmann L, Moergeli H, Creutzig J, Schnyder U. 2009. Mutual influence of PTSD symptoms and chronic pain among injured accident survivors: A longitudinal study. *Journal of Traumatic Stress*. 22(6):540–549.

Jensen M, Turner J, Romano J. 2000. Pain belief assessment: A comparison of the short and long versions of the Survey of Pain Attitudes. *The Journal of Pain*. 1(2):138–150.

Jensen MP. 2003. The validity and reliability of pain measures for use in clinical trials in adults. Presented at the second meeting of the initiative on Methods, Measurement, and Pain Assessment in Clinical Trials (IMMPACT-II); April 2003. Avaliable at: www.immpact.org/meetings.html. Acessed Aug 5, 2011.

Jensen MP, Karoly P. 2001. Self-report scales and procedures for assessing pain in adults. In: Turk DC, Melzack R, editors. *Handbook of Pain Assessment*, 2nd edition. New York: Guilford Press. 15–34.

Jensen MP, Turner JA, Romano JM. 1994. Relationship of pain specific beliefs to chronic pain adjustment. *Pain*. 57:301–309.

Katz J, Asmundson GJG, McRae K, et al. 2009. Emotional numbing and pain intensity predict the development of pain disability up to one year after lateral thoracotomy: a prospective, longitudinal cohort study. *European Journal of Pain* 13:870–878.

Keller S, Bann C, Dodd S, et al. 2004. Validity of the brief pain inventory for use in documenting the outcomes of patients with noncancer pain. *The Clinical Journal of Pain*. 20(5):309–318.

Kessler RC, Berglund PA, Bruce ML, et al. 2001. The prevalence and correlates of untreated serious mental illness. *Health Services Research*. 36:987–1007.

Kerns RD, Turk DC, Rudy TE. 1985. The West Haven-Yale Multidimenstional Pain Inventory (WHYMPI). *Pain*. 23:345–356.

Kerns RD, Rosengerg R, Jamison RN, et al. 1997. Readiness to adopt a self-management approach to chronic pain: The Pain Stages of Change Questionniare (PSOCQ). *Pain*. 72:227–234.

Kerns RD, Otis J, Rosenberg R, et al. 2003. Veterans' reports of pain and associations with ratings of health risk behaviors: Affective distress and use of the healthcare system. *Journal of Rehabilitation Research and Development*. 40:371–379.

Kiecolt-Glaser J, McGuire L, Robles T, et al. 2002. Psychoneuroimmunology: Psychological influences on immune function and health. Journal of Consulting and Clinical Psychology. 70(3):537–547.

Kraus A, Geuze E, Schmahl C, et al. 2009. Differentiation of pain ratings in combat-related posttraumatic stress disorder. Pain. 143:179–185.

Kuhn E. 2004. Peritraumatic risk factors and early posttraumatic maintaining factors of posttraumatic stress disorder in motor vehicle accident survivors. Dissertation Abstracts: AAT 3148023.

Lang PJ. 1979. A bioinformational theory of emotional imagery. Psychophysiology. 52: 1048–1060.

Lanius R, Bluhm R., Lanius U, et al. 2005. A review of neuroimaging studies in PTSD: Heterogeneity of response to symptom provocation. Journal of Psychiatric Research. 40:709–729.

Lariviere WR, Melzack R. 2000. The role of corticotropin-releasing factor in pain and analgesia. Pain. 84(1):1–12. (DOI: S0304-3959(99)00193-1 [pii]).

Liedl A, O'Donnell M, Creamer M, et al. 2010. Support for the mutual maintenance of pain and post-traumatic stress disorder symptoms. Psychological Medicine. 40:1215–1223.

McBeth J, Silman A J, Gupta A, et al. 2007. Moderation of psychosocial risk factors through dysfunction of the hypothalamic-pituitary-adrenal stress axis in the onset of chronic widespread musculoskeletal pain: findings of a population-based prospective cohort study. Arthritis Rheum. 56(1):360–371. (DOI: 10.1002/art.22336).

McEwen BS, Stellar E. 1993. Stress and the individual: Mechanisms leading to disease. Archives of Internal Medicine. 153:2093–2101.

McLean SA, Clauw DJ, Abelson JL, et al. 2005. The development of persistent pain and psychological morbidity after motor vehicle collision: integrating the potential role of stress response systems into a biopsychosocial model. Psychosom Med. 67(5):783–790. (DOI: 67/5/783 [pii] 10.1097/01.psy.0000181276.49204.bb).

Martin A, Halket E, Asmundson G, et al. 2010. Posttraumatic stress symptoms and the diathesis-stress model of chronic pain and disability in patients undergoing major surgery. The Clinical Journal of Pain. 26(6):518–527.

Melzak R. 1987. The Short-Form McGuill Pain Questionaire. Pain. 30(2):191–197.

Melzak R, Katz J. 2004. The Gate-Control Theory: reaching for the brain. In: Hadjistavropoulos T, Craig KD, editors. *Pain: Psychological Perspectives*. Mahwah, NJ: Lawrence Erlbaum Associates. 13–34.

Nielson WR, Armstrong JM, Jensen MP, et al. 2009. Two brief versions of the Multidimensional Pain Readiness to Change Questionnaire, Version 2 (MPRCQ2). *The Clinical Journal of Pain*. 25(1):48–57.

Nielson WR, Jensen, MP, Kerns RD. 2003. Initial development and validation of a Multidimensional Pain Readiness to Change Questionnaire (MPRCQ). *Journal of Pain*. 4:148–158.

Ng KF, Tsui SL, Chan WS. 2002. Prevalence of common chronic pain in Hong Kong adults. *Clinical Journal of Pain*. 18:275–281.

Norman SB, Stein MB, Dimsdale JE, et al. 2007. Pain in the aftermath of trauma is a risk factor for post-traumatic stress disorder. *Psychological Medicine*. 38:533–542.

Osman A, Barrios F, Gutierrez P, et al. 2000. The pain catastrophizing scale: further psychometric evaluation with adult samples. *Journal of Behavioral Medicine*. 23(4):351–356.

Otis JD. 2007. *Managing Chronic Pain: A Cognitive-Behavioral Approach*. New York: Oxford University Press.

Otis JD, Gregor K, Hardway C, et al. 2010. An examination of the comorbidity between chronic pain and posttraumatic stress disorder on U.S. Veterans. *Psychological Services*. 7(3):126–135.

Otis JD, Keane TM, Kerns RD. 2003. An examination of the relationship between chronic pain and Posttraumatic Stress Disorder. *Journal of Rehabilitation, Research, and Development*. 40(5):397–406.

Otis JD, Keane, TM, Kerns RD, et al. 2009. The development of an integrated treatment for veterans with comorbid chronic pain and posttraumatic stress disorder. *Pain Medicine*. 10(7):1300–1311.

Otis JD, Pincus DB, Keane T. 2006. Comorbid chronic pain and posttraumatic stress disorder across the lifespan: a review of theoretical models. In: Young G, Kane AW, Nicholson K, editors. *Psychological Knowledge in Court*. New York: Springer, 242–268.

O'Toole BI, Catts SV. 2008. Trauma, PTSD, and physical health: an epidemiological study of Australian Vietnam veterans. *J Psychosom Res*. 64(1):33–40. (DOI: S0022-3999(07)00289-9 [pii] 10.1016/j.jpsychores.2007.07.006).

Patterson DR, Tininenko J, Ptacek JT. 2006. Pain during hospitalization predicts long-term outcome. *Journal of Burn Care and Research.* 27(5):719–726.

Paylo SA, Beck JG. 2005. Post-traumatic stress disorder symptoms, pain, and perceived life control: Associations with psychosocial and physical functioning. *Pain.* 117:121–127.

Pitman R, Orr S, vander Kolk B, et al. 1990. Analgesia: A new dependent variable for the biological study of posttraumatic stress disorder. In: Wolf M, Mosnaim A, editors. *Posttraumatic Stress Disorder: Etiology, phenomenology, and treatment.* Washington DC: American Psychiatric Association.

Ploghaus A, Becerra L, Borras C, et al. 2003. Neural circuitry underlying pain modulation: Expectation, hypnosis, placebo. *Trends in Cognitive Sciences.*, 7(5):197–200.

Poundja J, Fikretoglu D, Brunet A. 2006. The co-occurrence of posttraumatic stress disorder symptoms and pain: Is depression a mediator. *Journal of Traumatic Stress.* 19(5):747–751.

Resick PA, Monson CM, Chard KM. 2007. *Cognitive processing therapy: Veteran/ military version.* Washington, DC: Department of Veterans' Affairs.

Resnick H S, Kilpatrick DG, Dansky BS, et al. 1993. Prevalence of civilian trauma and posttraumatic stress disorder in a representative national sample of women. *Journal of Consulting and Clinical Psychology.* 61:984–991.

Roth RS, Geisser ME, Bates R. 2008. The relation of post-traumatic stress symptoms to depression and pain in patients with accident-related chronic pain. *The Journal of Pain.* 97:588–596.

Rustoen T, Wahl, AK, Hanestad BR, et al. 2004. Gender differences in chronic pain—Findings from a population-based study of Norwegian adults. *Pain Management Nursing: Official Journal of the American Society of Pain Management Nurses.* 5(3):105–117.

Saltzman LE, Fanslow JL, McMahon PM, et al. 1999. Intimate partner violence surveillance: Uniform definitions and recommended data elements. Atlanta, GA: Centers for Disease Control and Prevention.

Sareen J, Cox B, Stein M, et al. 2007. Physical and mental comorbidity, disability, and suicidal behavior associated with posttraumatic stress disorder in a large community sample. *Psychosomatic Medicine.* 69:242–248.

Saxe G, Stoddard F, Courtney D, et al. 2001. Relationship between acute morphine and the course of PTSD in children with burns. *American Academy of Child and Adolescent Psychiatry.* 40(8).

Schnurr PP, Friedman MJ, Sengupta A, et al. 2000. *Journal of Nervous and Mental Disease.* 188(8):496–504.

Schnurr PP, Green BL, editors, 2004. *Trauma and Health: Physical Health Consequences of Exposure to Extreme Stress.* Washington, DC: American Psychological Association.

Sharp TJ, Harvey AG. 2001. Chronic pain and posttraumatic stress disorder: Mutual Maintenance? *Clinical Psychology Review.* 21:857–877.

Sherbourne C, Asch SM, Shugarman LR, et al. 2009. Early identification of co-occurring pain, depression, and anxiety. *Journal of General Internal Medicine.* 24(5):620–625.

Shipherd JC. 2006. Treatment of a case example with PTSD and chronic pain. *Cognitive and Behavioral Practice.* 13:24–32.

Shipherd JC, Beck JG, Hamblen JL, et al. 2003. A preliminary examination of treatment for Posttraumatic Stress Disorder in chronic pain patients: A case study. *Journal of Traumatic Stress.* 16(5):451–457.

Shipherd JC, Keyes M, Jovanovic T, et al. 2007. Veterans seeking treatment for posttraumatic stress disorder: What about comorbid chronic pain? *Journal of Rehabilitation Research and Development.* 44(2):153–166.

Sledjeski EM, Speisman B, Dierker LC. 2008. Does number of lifetime traumas explain the relationship between PTSD and chronic medical conditions? Answers from the National Comorbidity Survey Replication (NSC-R). *Journal of Behavior Medicine.* 31:341–349.

Sterling M, Jull G, Vicenzino B, et al. 2005. Physical and psychological factors predict outcome following whiplash injury, Pain, 114, 141–148.

Sterling M, Kenardy J. 2006. The relationship between sensory and sympathetic nervous system changes and posttraumatic stress reaction following whiplash injury—a prospective study. *Journal of Psychosomatic Research.* 60:387–393.

Sterling M, Kenardy J, Jull G, et al. 2003. The development of psychological changes following whiplash injury. *Pain.* 106:481–489.

Strigo I, Simmons A, Matthews S, et al. 2010. Neural correlates of altered pain response in women with posttraumatic stress disorder from intimate partner violence. *Biological Psychiatry.* 68:442–450.

Sullivan M, Bishop S, Picik J. 1995. The pain catastrophizing scale: development and validation. *Psychological Assessment.* 7(4):524–532.

Taylor S, Fedoroff I, Koch W, et al. 2001. Posttraumatic stress disorder arising after road traffic collisions: Patters of response to cognitive-behavior therapy. *Journal of Consulting and Clinical Psychology.* 69(3):541–551.

Thorn BE. 2004. *Cognitive Therapy for Chronic Pain.* New York: The Guildford Press.

Tanriverdi F, Karaca Z, Unluhizarci K, et al. 2007. The hypothalamo-pituitary-adrenal axis in chronic fatigue syndrome and fibromyalgia syndrome. *Stress.* 10(1):13–25. (DOI: 773423011 [pii] 10.1080/10253890601130823).

Turk DC, Okifuji A. 1996. Perception of traumatic onset, compensation status, and physical findings: Impact on pain severity, emotional distress, and disability in chronic pain patients. *Journal of Behavioral Medicine.* 19:435–453.

Turk DD, Okifuji A. 2002. Psychological factors in chronic pain: Evolution and revolution. *Journal of Consulting and Clinical Psychology.* 70(3):678–690.

Vierck CJ, Jr. 2006. Mechanisms underlying development of spatially distributed chronic pain (fibromyalgia). *Pain.* 124(3):242–263. (DOI: S0304-3959(06)00308-3 [pii]).

Von Korff M, Crane P, Lane M, et al. 2005. Chronic spinal pain and physical-mental comorbidity in the United States: Results from the national comorbidity survey replication. *Pain.* 113:331–339.

Van Loey NEE, Maas CJM, Faber AW, et al. 2003. Predictors of chronic posttraumatic stress symptoms following burn injury: results of a longitudinal study. *Journal of Traumatic Stress.* 16(4):361–369.

Von Korff M, Dworkin SF, LeResche L. 1990. Graded chronic pain status: an epidemiologic evaluation. *Pain.* 40:279–291.

Weisberg R, Bruce S, Machan J, et al. 2002. Nonpsychiatric illness among primary care patients with trauma histories and posttraumatic stress disorder. *Psychiatric Services.* 53(7):848–854.

Williams DA, Thorn BE. 1989. An empirical assessment of pain beliefs. *Pain*. 36:351–358.

Wald J, Taylor S, Chiri, LR, et al. 2010. Posttraumatic stress disorder and chronic pain arising from motor vehicle accidents: Efficacy of interoceptive exposure plus trauma-related exposure therapy. *Cognitive Behaviour Therapy*. 39(2):104–113.

Wald J. 2008. Interoceptive exposure as a prelude to trauma-related exposure therapy in a case of Posttraumatic Stress Disorder with substantial comorbidity. *Journal of Cognitive Psychotherapy: An International Quarterly*. 22(4):331–345.

Wuest J, Ford-Gilboe M, Merritt-Gray M, et al. 2009. Abuse-related injury and symptoms of Posttraumatic Stress Disorder as mechanisms of chronic pain in survivors of intimate partner violence. *Pain Medicine*. 10(4):739–747.

Wuest J, Ford-Gilboe M, Merritt-Gray M, et al. 2010. Pathways of chronic pain in survivors of intimate partner violence. *Journal of Women's Health*. 19(9):1665–1674.

Yehuda R. 2006. Advances in understanding neuroendocrine alterations in PTSD and their therapeutic implications. *Ann N Y Acad Sci*. 1071:137–2006.

6

Post-Traumatic Stress Disorder and Obesity, Diabetes, and the Metabolic Syndrome

Steven S. Coughlin, Ph.D., and Yasmin S. Cypel, Ph.D., M.S.

An increasing number of studies have examined the relationships between chronic stress and metabolic disorders such as obesity, diabetes, and the metabolic syndrome. Additional studies have examined the development of diabetes and obesity among persons with post-traumatic stress disorder (PTSD) who have had traumatic exposures during combat or civilian life, as reviewed later in this chapter. Associations between PTSD and the metabolic syndrome have also been reported (Heppner et al. 2009; Jin et al. 2009; Maslov et al. 2009; Rasmusson et al. 2010). The results of these studies indicate that important neurobiological and psychophysiological changes can occur among people suffering from PTSD as well as among healthy individuals who are exposed to chronic stress (McFarlane 2010). Through the brain, neurohormonal mediators, and the autonomic nervous system, stress can have acute and chronic affects on adipose and muscle tissues as well as the cardiovascular and immune systems (McEwen and Stellar 1993). Additionally, as detailed below, stress can result in elevations of cortisol and insulin.

PHYSIOLOGICAL BASIS OF THE STRESS RESPONSE: THE HYPOTHALAMIC-PITUITARY-ADRENAL AXIS SYSTEM AND GLUCOCORTICOIDS

The effects of traumatic exposures or chronic stress on the hypothalamic-pituitary-adrenal axis (HPA) and the autonomic nervous system have been examined in clinical studies and in animal models. In healthy adults, stress and anxiety have been associated with increased cortisol, plasma and urinary norepinephrine, epinephrine, and their metabolites (Lader 1974; Bedi and Arora 2007). Glucocorticoids, mainly cortisol in humans, are part of a class of steroid hormones called corticosteroids that are released by the adrenal cortex in response to adrenocorticotropic hormone (ACTH) produced in the anterior pituitary gland. The production and secretion of ACTH by the pituitary is stimulated by hypothalamic corticotropin-releasing hormone (CRH). This system of hormones is typically kept in balance through the existence of a negative feedback loop that acts to inhibit both CRH secretions by the hypothalamus and ACTH by the pituitary when threshold blood concentrations of cortisol are reached.

Clinical studies have found that cerebrospinal fluid levels of CRH are elevated in patients with PTSD, which is consistent with increased activity of the HPA system in the central nervous system (Bremner et al. 1997; Baker et al. 2005; Rohleder and Karl 2006). In studies of urinary cortisol excretion in patients with PTSD, urinary cortisol concentrations have been reported to be elevated in some but not all studies (Yehuda et al. 1993; Rohleder and Karl 2006).

The metabolic processes influenced by the release of corticosteroids include the formation of glucose from fatty acids and amino acids. Cortisol stimulates gluconeogenesis in the liver by increasing insulin insensitivity and enhancing the expression of enzymes involved in gluconeogenesis. Cortisol also inhibits the uptake of glucose in adipose and muscle tissues and stimulates the breakdown of fats in adipose tissue. Sustained elevations of cortisol can lead to hyperlipidemia (McEwen and Stellar 1993). Corticosteroids also have regulatory effects on the immune system as noted in Chapter 1.

PHYSIOLOGICAL AND SYMPTOMATIC RELATIONSHIP AMONG OBESITY, DIABETES, AND METABOLIC SYNDROME

The metabolic syndrome, which is a major risk factor for type 2 diabetes mellitus and cardiovascular disease, encompasses several metabolic and physiological disturbances including dyslipidemia, hyperglycemia, hypertension, obesity (Giovannucci and Michaud 2007), and the proinflammatory state (Reilly and Rader 2003). In the United States and many other developed countries, the metabolic syndrome affects about one-quarter of adults over the age of 20, and as many as 45% of those over the age of 50 years (Reilly and Rader 2003). The dyslipidemias seen in metabolic syndrome include high concentrations of serum triglycerides, very low-density lipoprotein (VLDL) cholesterol, and low-density lipoprotein (LDL) cholesterol and low concentrations of high-density lipoprotein (HDL) cholesterol. Chronic inflammation, procoagulation, and impaired fibrinolysis have also been associated with the syndrome. Like most chronic conditions, the etiology of metabolic syndrome is multifactorial and only partly understood. Obesity (particularly abdominal or visceral adiposity), physical inactivity, and insulin resistance are among the underlying factors for this syndrome. Elevated body mass index (BMI), abdominal or visceral adiposity, and physical inactivity are the major modifiable risk factors for insulin resistance, the metabolic syndrome, and hyperinsulinemia (Giovannucci and Michaud 2007).

Hyperinsulinemia is one of the early manifestations of disease for individuals with diabetes mellitus, although insulin concentrations eventually decrease due to pancreatic beta cell depletion (Giovannucci and Michaud 2007). Hyperinsulinemia has been hypothesized to be an underlying factor in chronic conditions such as obesity, type 2 diabetes mellitus, and certain forms of cancer. Obesity and physical inactivity are important determinants of hyperinsulinemia and insulin resistance in the non-diabetic state (Giovannucci and Michaud 2007). Insulin levels are higher in diabetics and in obese persons. Several metabolic imbalances including hyperglycemia and hypertriglyceridemia are associated with hyperinsulinemia and insulin resistance.

CHRONIC STRESS, OBESITY AND THE METABOLIC SYNDROME

In the absence of dietary changes or reduced physical activity, chronic stress can lead to weight loss through adrenergic activation. However, weight gain may occur in response to stress, which may be due to an increased intake of high-fat and high-sugar "comfort foods" (Dallman et al. 2003; Kuo et al. 2008). There may be additional biological mechanisms by which chronic stress leads to insulin resistance and the metabolic syndrome. Although glucocorticoids act peripherally to mobilize energy stores in adipose tissue and muscle for use in hepatic gluconeogenesis, animal studies have shown that they also act centrally in the brain to motivate caloric intake and to augment learning and behaviors associated with increased food intake of fat-enriched foods (Dallman et al.

2007). Stress-induced elevations in glucocorticoids may promote food intake and obesity through emotion-mediated brain networks (Dallman 2010).

Several epidemiologic and clinical studies have examined obesity and the metabolic syndrome as possible consequences of chronic stress (Chrousos and Gold 1992; Rasmusson et al. 2010). In a double-blind case-control study in Great Britain, which examined working men aged 45–63 from the Whitehall II cohort (Marmot and Brunner 2005), Brunner et al. (2002) observed associations between metabolic syndrome and physiological markers of stress-related neuroendocrine and autonomic activation (low heart rate variability, elevated cortisol levels, and higher levels of interleukin-6). More recent analyses of data from the Whitehall II cohort have suggested a dose-response relationship between occupational stress and the metabolic syndrome (Chandola et al. 2006). Chronic stress has also been associated with obesity and the metabolic syndrome in an animal model in which mice were exposed to both stressors and a high-fat/high-sugar diet (Kuo et al. 2008).

PTSD, TRAUMATIC EXPERIENCE, AND OBESITY

An increasing number of studies in the United States and other countries have identified weight change and obesity as important health concerns among persons of various ages who were exposed to traumatic experiences (Das et al. 2005; Kress et al. 2005; Wang et al. 2005; Trief et al. 2006; Nelson 2006; Almond et al. 2008). The association between PTSD and obesity has been reported in several veteran populations (Cohen et al. 2009a; Heppner et al. 2009; Chwastiak et al. 2011) although not all studies have found this association (Barber et al. 2011). The biological pathways that underlie these associations may relate to the HPA system and biological responses to chronic anxiety and stress. Taking into account evidence from studies conducted in the general population, persons who are overweight or obese are likely to be at increased risk for adult-onset chronic diseases such as coronary heart disease, diabetes, arthritis, and several forms of cancer (Yarnell et al. 2000; Calle 2007; Byun et al. 2010).

Due to military training and the physical demands of war, military personnel and recent veterans tend to be physically fit. However, as cohorts of veterans advance in age (for example, U.S. veterans who served in the 1990–1991 Gulf War), they are likely to be at risk of not only certain deployment-related health conditions (for example, PTSD), but also obesity and other chronic conditions.

Dobie et al. (2004) surveyed women (n = 1,935) who received care at the Department of Veterans Affairs Puget Sound Health Care System between October 1996 and January 1998. The survey included questions about medical history and health habits. The PTSD Checklist-Civilian Version (PCL-C) was included. Of the 1,259 eligible women who completed the survey, 266 (21%) screened positive for current PTSD (PCL-C score $\geq$ 50). Based upon self-reported height and weight, women with PTSD were more likely to be obese (age-adjusted odds ratio = 1.78; 95% confidence interval 1.34–2.35). Obesity was defined as a BMI (kg/m^2) > 30.

Cohen et al. (2009a) examined associations between PTSD and obesity and other cardiovascular risk factors among Operation Enduring Freedom and Operation Iraqi Freedom (OEF/OIF) veterans who sought care at VA health care facilities. Veterans with mental health diagnoses had a significantly higher frequency of obesity. For example, among 65,603 male OEF/OIF veterans who had PTSD with or without other mental health diagnoses, the adjusted odds ratio for the association between PTSD and obesity was 2.35 (95% confidence interval 2.27–2.43) after controlling for age, race/ethnicity (white, black, Hispanic, or other), military component type (active duty vs. National Guard/ Reserve), rank, branch of service, and multiple deployments. Among 6,964 female OEF/OIF veterans who had PTSD with or without other mental health diagnoses, the adjusted odds ratio for the association between PTSD and obesity was 3.01 (95% confidence interval 2.76–3.28) after controlling for the same set of predictors.

Coughlin et al. (2011) examined relationships between PTSD, obesity, and symptom-based health conditions (chronic fatigue syndrome-like illness and unexplained multisymptom illness). The data used was from a cross-sectional survey of health information among population-based samples of 15,000 veterans of the 1991 Gulf War and 15,000 veterans who served during the same era (Coughlin et al. 2011). Data were collected from 9,970 respondents in 2003–2005 via a structured mail questionnaire or telephone survey. Based on BMI (kg/ m^2) estimated from self-reported information about height and weight, the percentages of Gulf War (n = 6,111) and Gulf Era veterans (n = 3,859) who were overweight (25 $\leq$ BMI $\leq$ 29.9), were 46.8% and 48.7%, respectively. The percentage of the veterans who were obese (BMI $\geq$ 30) were 29.6% and 28.3%, respectively. Without adjustment for Gulf deployment status (Gulf War versus Gulf Era), age, sex, or other factors; PTSD, unexplained multi-symptom illness, and chronic fatigue syndrome (CFS)-like illness were more common among obese veterans than those who were normal weight ($18.5 \leq BMI \leq 24.9$). The odds ratio for the association between PTSD and obesity was 1.4 (95% confidence interval 1.2–1.7). This association remained statistically significant (adjusted odds ratio = 1.5, 95% confidence interval 1.2–1.8) when CFS-like illness and unexplained multisymptom illness were added to the model.

Vieweg et al. (2006a) addressed the prevalence of obesity in 252 male veterans who had clinical features of PTSD and attended the PTSD program at the Department of Veterans Affairs Medical Center (VAMC) in Richmond, Virginia. Investigators found that 84.1% of these men were overweight ($25 \leq BMI < 30$), obese ($30 \leq BMI < 40$), or morbidly obese ($BMI \geq 40$); approximately 46.4% were obese or morbidly obese. The prevalence of obesity ($BMI \geq 25$) was greater than age-adjusted, nationally based estimates for men aged 20 years or older (Flegal et al. 2002). In another analysis based on veterans from the same VAMC, similar conclusions were reached (Vieweg et al. 2006b). Additional research suggested that the BMI of male veterans with PTSD was significantly greater ($p < 0.0001$) than the BMI of veterans without PTSD (Vieweg et al. 2007). Kress et al. (2006) found that the odds of depressive symptoms in obese men and women, who were active duty military service personnel, were greater than those of normal-weight individuals.

The troops who served in the 1991 Gulf War were exposed to many stressors including rapid mobilization, war-time hostilities, and concerns about potential chemical attacks. These and other war-time exposures (for example, witnessing deaths or being exposed to hostile fire) may have led to PTSD among some of these veterans. Although speculative, it is possible that veterans with PTSD are more likely to consume a high caloric diet, exercise less, and have other unhealthy lifestyle behaviors that may lead to obesity and other disorders. The relationship between health behaviors and PTSD is an important area of future study.

PTSD AND DIABETES

Persons with PTSD are more likely to have diabetes mellitus in epidemiologic and clinical studies as compared with persons without PTSD (Weisberg et al.

2002; Boscarino 2004; David et al. 2004; Kimerling 2004). Potential biological mechanisms for a link between PTSD and diabetes include insulin resistance resulting from circulating mediators of inflammation (e.g., cytokines/ interleukins). Changes in immune function reported in PTSD patients include higher levels of interleukins in the blood (Spivak et al. 1997; Maes et al. 1999; Tucker et al. 2004; Rohleder and Karl 2006).

Table 6.1 presents findings from studies that examine PTSD and diabetes. Some studies suggest a positive association between PTSD and diabetes, although other studies have not found this association (Schnurr et al. 2000a; Norman et al. 2006).

PTSD AND THE METABOLIC SYNDROME

Metabolic syndrome is manifested by a number of conditions including dyslipidemia, chronic inflammation, and hypertension (Reilly and Rader 2003; Giovannucci 2007). Kibler et al. (2009) found that the prevalence of hypertension was higher in individuals with PTSD (with or without depression) relative to those with depression only ($p < 0.05$) or those with no mental illness ($p < 0.001$), using data collected from civilians in the 1990–1992 National Comorbidity Survey. Hypertension was also evident in Australian Vietnam veterans with PTSD (O'Toole and Catts 2008) and in World War II prisoners of war with PTSD (Kang et al. 2006). Hypertension and other measures of allostatic load, including serum lipids and glycosylated hemoglobin, are recognized as important physiological factors in individuals with PTSD (Bedi and Arora 2007; Kibler 2009; Dedert et al. 2010). Studies have demonstrated the existence of various combinations of these conditions in PTSD-afflicted individuals (Schnurr et al. 2000a, 2000b; Weisberg et al. 2002; David et al. 2004; Dobie et al. 2004; Kimerling 2004; Lauterbach et al. 2005). Stress-induced disruption of the HPA system has also been associated with glucose metabolism disorders in an animal model of PTSD (Cohen et al. 2009b).

The metabolic syndrome has been specifically studied in relation to PTSD. Factors associated with the metabolic syndrome have been examined in clinical studies of persons with PTSD (Heppner et al. 2009; Jin et al. 2009). Heppner et al. (2009) examined data from 253 male and female veterans, of whom 139 (55%) met Diagnostic and Statistical Manual of Mental Disorders, fourth edition (DSM-IV) criteria for PTSD. The variables examined in their analysis

Table 6.1. Studies of PTSD and Diabetes Among Various Populations

Study	Sample	Study Design/Objective	Results	Limitations	Other Information
Boscarino 2004	2,490 male Vietnam veterans	Data obtained from Vietnam Experience Study (VES).[1] Telephone survey, medical examination with personal interviews, and mortality analysis. Data obtained from phase 3 of the VES; latter collected mainly in 1986. Objective was to examine association between chronic PTSD and common autoimmune diseases.	Chronic Post-Traumatic Stress Disorder (PTSD) is associated with common autoimmune conditions including insulin-dependent diabetes, rheumatoid arthritis, psoriasis, and thyroid disease.	Disease outcomes based partially on self-report may be problematic. Study was based only on men.	Large-scale population study; random sample obtained.
Boyko et al. 2010	Millennium Cohort Study of male and female U.S. military service members who completed baseline and follow-up questionnaires. Of these, data for 44,378 were used for analysis.	Self-administered survey, data also linked to Department of Defense (DoD) databases. Objective was to examine the relationship between diabetes risk and combat deployment/mental health.	After adjustment for age, sex, body mass index, education, race/ethnicity, military service characteristics, and mental health conditions, baseline PTSD was significantly associated with diabetes risk.	Outcomes were self-reported. No validation. PTSD medications could have contributed to development of diabetes.	Prospective investigation of the association between PTSD and diabetes and other outcomes.

(continued on next page)

Table 6.1. (*continued*)

Study	Sample	Study Design/Objective	Results	Limitations	Other Information
David et al. 2004	Male veterans recruited from rehabilitation unit in Miami Veterans Affairs Medical Center for chronic PTSD (n=55) or alcohol dependence (n=38).	Mental health interviews, structured interview for health habits, medical history, and physical exam (included laboratory tests, imaging studies). Objective was to examine prevalence of specific health problems and health risk factors.	Diabetes and heart disease were more frequent among patients with PTSD.	Possible over-reporting of symptoms. Small sample size. Results may not be generalized to other veterans, given subjects had severe PTSD and alcohol dependence.	Aging population of veterans may be more at risk of specific medical condition.
Kimerling 2004	Sample obtained from non-institutionalized civilian population, n=5,877 [men (n=2835), women (n=3042)]–National Comorbidity Survey (NCS)[2].	Objective was to examine non-psychiatric illnesses associated with PTSD. Focus on multiple disorders, including diabetes.	PTSD was associated with an increased likelihood of diabetes among women (adjusted OR=2.2, 95% CI 1.1–4.8). Among men, PTSD was not associated with an increased likelihood of diabetes.	Sample restricted to relatively healthy individuals – no elderly or persons in institutions. Timeline of outcome occurrence relative to PTSD is not known.	Multistage survey of the civilian population representing the 48 contiguous states.

(continued on next page)

Table 6.1. (*continued*)

Study	Sample	Study Design/Objective	Results	Limitations	Other Information
Lauterbach et al. 2005	Sample obtained from non-institutionalized civilian population, n=5,877 [with lifetime history of PTSD, n=429 (weighted); no PTSD, n=5448] – NCS^2.	To examine relationship between PTSD and self-reported health problems. Focus on multiple disorders, including diabetes.	Individuals with lifetime history of PTSD were at increased risk to report diabetes ($\chi = 7.90$, $p < 0.01$).	Data were self-reported; limited to civilian population; PTSD group is heterogeneous regarding recovery status.	Multistage survey of the civilian population representing the 48 contiguous states.
Norman et al. 2006	n=680 primary care patients (421 women, 259 men).	Telephone interview administered CIDI, self-administered questionnaire on physical illness and demographics.	Although trauma was associated with significant increases in the odds for diabetes in men, PTSD was not related to diabetes. No association found in women for trauma, diabetes, and PTSD.	Timing of physical problems relative to trauma and PTSD; bias resulting from systematic sampling; assessment of only current PTSD; small number of observations for certain illnesses with loss of power.	Trauma may be an important factor in the examination of the association between PTSD and physical health.

(continued on next page)

Table 6.1. (continued)

Study	Sample	Study Design/Objective	Results	Limitations	Other Information
Weisberg et al. 2002	n=502 primary care patients with 1 or more anxiety disorders	Self-administered current/lifetime health questionnaire; assessment of diagnostic criteria (Structured Clinical Interview for DSM-IV) for one or more index disorders (including PTSD).	Highest rates of diabetes were reported by the PTSD group and lowest by participants with no trauma history. Logistic regression showed only that age was significantly ($p < 0.05$) related to diabetes while controlling for other covariates including PTSD.	Self-reported data on physical illnesses.	Longitudinal research needed to assess how PTSD improvement relates to reduction in associated comorbid conditions.
Schnurr et al. 2000a	n=250 Army and n=250 Navy male veterans; randomly selected from Department of Veterans Affairs mortality study registry.	Telephone interviews (CATI) on mustard gas testing, PTSD, lifetime trauma, current health, and demographics. Diabetes was one of many illnesses examined in relation to PTSD status.	There was no association between full or partial PTSD with self-reported diabetes.	Self-reported data. No use of objective measures such as physician diagnosis or laboratory exams. Unable to establish temporal relationship between PTSD and health outcomes.	Relatively large sample.

[1] CDC 1988a, 1988b

[2] Kessler et al. 1994

included systolic and diastolic blood pressure, waist-to-hip ratio, and fasting measures of HDL cholesterol, serum triglycerides, and plasma glucose concentration. After controlling for several demographic factors such as alcohol use, substance abuse, smoking, and depression, PTSD severity was a significant predictor (p = 0.03) of metabolic syndrome status. After assessment, metabolic syndrome status was defined as satisfaction of three or more of the following five criteria: (1) elevated serum triglycerides; (2) blood pressure; (3) waist-to-hip ratio; (4) plasma glucose concentration; and (5) decreased HDL. In another study, police officers diagnosed with severe PTSD showed a significantly increased prevalence (prevalence ratio = 3.31, 95% confidence interval 1.19–9.22) of metabolic syndrome compared to those with the least severe PTSD status (Violanti et al. 2006). Other studies suggest consideration of other comorbid physical and mental disorders when investigating PTSD and metabolic syndrome (Jakovljevic et al. 2006, 2008; Babic et al. 2007; Maslov et al. 2009).

SUMMARY AND CONCLUSIONS

Further research is needed to better understand the complex relationships surrounding PTSD and comorbidities such as obesity, diabetes, and metabolic syndrome. This is well illustrated in a multifactorial PTSD outcome model proposed by Boscarino (2004) where heredity, behavior, trauma exposure, and biological alterations comprise just a few of the relevant factors requiring consideration. The establishment of consensus regarding causal relationships is difficult because insufficient numbers of prospective studies have been completed to date, which weakens evidence for temporally based patterns. Long-term prospective research may provide further information about how currently utilized PTSD treatment strategies could reduce the comorbid conditions associated with this disorder (Weisberg et al. 2002). More research should target different demographic groups. Many studies have focused on men. Further study also needs to consider greater validation of the self-reported health outcome data that has been frequently relied upon to draw conclusions about possible associations. Validation approaches could include physician-confirmed diagnoses or medical record reviews to help substantiate reported data. Although this review may not have been exhaustive, the challenge facing most researchers in the compilation of findings was evident, given differences in the type and number of covariates controlled for, statistical methods, manner of PTSD diagnosis, target group characteristics, sample size, and the manner in which physical outcomes were defined. The identification of biomarkers may represent another approach for the improved understanding of PTSD and co-occurring conditions.

REFERENCES

Almond N, Kahwati L, Kinsinger L, et al. 2008. The prevalence of overweight and obesity among U.S. military veterans. *Mil Med.* 173:544–549.

Babic D, Jakovljevic M, Martinac M, et al. 2007. Metabolic syndrome and combat posttraumatic stress disorder intensity: preliminary findings. *Psychiatr Danub.* 19:68–75.

Baker DG, Ekhator NN, Kasckow JW, et al. 2005. Higher levels of basal serial CSF cortisol in combat veterans with posttraumatic stress disorder. *Am J Psychiatry.* 162:992–994.

Barber J, Bayer L, Pietrzak RH, Sanders KA. 2011. Assessment of rates of overweight and obesity and symptoms of posttraumatic stress disorder and depression in a sample of Operation Enduring Freedom/Operation Iraqi Freedom veterans. *Mil Med.* 176:151–155.

Bedi US, Arora R. 2007. Cardiovascular manifestations of posttraumatic stress disorder. *J Natl Med Assoc.* 99:642–649.

Boscarino JA. 2004. Posttraumatic stress disorder and physical illness. Results from clinical and epidemiologic studies. *Ann NY Acad Sci.* 1032:141–153.

Boyko EJ, Jacobson IG, Smith B, et al. 2010. Risk of diabetes in U.S. military service members in relation to combat deployment and mental health. *Diabetes Care.* 33:1771–1777.

Bremner JD, Licinio J, Darnell A, et al. 1997. Elevated CSF corticotropin-releasing factor concentrations in posttraumatic stress disorder. *Am J Psychiatry.* 154:624–629.

Brunner EJ, Hemingway H, Walker BR, et al. 2002. Adrenocortical, autonomic, and inflammatory causes of the metabolic syndrome: nested case-control study. *Circulation.* 106:2659–2665.

Byun W, Sieverdes JC, Sui X, et al. 2010. Effect of positive health factors and all-cause mortality in men. *Med Sci Sports Exerc.* 42:1632–1638.

Calle E. 2007. Obesity and cancer. *BMJ.* 335:1107–1108.

Centers for Disease Control. 1988a. Health status of Vietnam veterans: I. Psychosocial characteristics. The Centers for Disease Control Vietnam Experience Study. *JAMA.* 259:2701–2707.

Centers for Disease Control. 1988b. Health status of Vietnam veterans: II. Physical health. The Centers for Disease Control Vietnam Experience Study. *JAMA.* 259:2708–2714.

Chandola T, Brunner E, Marmot M. 2006. Chronic stress at work and the metabolic syndrome: prospective study. *BMJ.* 332:521–525.

Chrousos GP, Gold PW. 1992. The concepts of stress and stress system disorders. Overview of physical and behavioral homeostasis. *JAMA.* 267:1244–1252.

Chwastiak LA, Rosenheck RA, Kazis LE. 2011. Association of psychiatric illness and obesity, physical inactivity, and smoking among a national sample of veterans. *Psychosomatics.* 52:230–236.

Cohen BE, Marmar C, Ren L, et al. 2009. Association of cardiovascular risk factors with mental health diagnoses in Iraq and Afghanistan War Veterans using VA health care. *JAMA.* 302:489–492.

Cohen H, Kozlovsky N, Savion N, et al. 2009. An association between stress-induced disruption of the hypothalamic-pituitary-adrenal axis and disordered glucose metabolism in an animal model of post-traumatic stress disorder. *J Neuroendocrinol.* 21:898–909.

Coughlin SS, Kang HK, Mahan CM. 2011. Selected health conditions among overweight, obese, and non-obese veterans of the 1991 Gulf War: Results from a survey conducted in 2003–2005. *The Open Epidemiology Journal.* 4:140–146.

Dallman MF, Pecoraro N, Akana SF, et al. 2003. Chronic stress and obesity: a new view of "comfort food." *Proc Natl Acad Sci USA.* 100:11696–11701.

Dallman MF, Warne JP, Foster MT, et al. 2007. Glucocorticoids and insulin both modulate caloric intake through actions on the brain. *J Physiol.* 583:431–436.

Dallman MF. 2010. Stress-induced obesity and the emotional nervous system. *Trends Endocrinol Metab.* 21:159–165.

Das SR, Kinsinger LS, Yancy WS Jr., et al. 2005. Obesity prevalence among veterans at Veterans Affairs medical facilities. *Am J Prev Med.* 28:291–294.

David D, Woodward C, Esquenazi J, et al. 2004. Comparison of comorbid physical illnesses among veterans with PTSD and veterans with alcohol dependence. *Psychiatr Serv.* 55:82–85.

Dedert EA, Calhoun PS, Watkins LL, et al. 2010. Posttraumatic stress disorder, cardiovascular, and metabolic disease: a review of the evidence. *Ann Behav Med.* 39:61–78.

Dobie DJ, Kivlahan DR, Maynard C., et al. 2004. Posttraumatic stress disorder in female veterans. Association with self-reported health problems and functional impairment. *Arch Intern Med.* 164:394–400.

Flegal KM, Carroll MD, Ogden CL, et al. 2002. Prevalence and trends in obesity among US adults, 1999–2000. *JAMA.* 288:1723–1727.

Giovannucci E, Michaud D. 2007. The role of obesity and related metabolic disturbances in cancers of the colon, prostate, and pancreas. *Gastroenterology.* 132:2208–2225.

Giovannucci E. 2007. Metabolic syndrome, hyperinsulinemia, and colon cancer: a review. *Am J Clin Nutr.* 86(suppl):836S–842S.

Heppner PS, Crawford EF, Haji UA, et al. 2009. The association of posttraumatic stress disorder and metabolic syndrome: a study of increased health risk in veterans. *BMC Med.* 7:1–8.

Jakovljevic M, Babic D, Crncevic Z, et al. 2008. Metabolic syndrome and depression in war veterans with posttraumatic stress disorder. *Psychiatr Danub.* 20:406–410.

Jakovljevic M, Saric M, Nad S, et al. 2006. Metabolic syndrome, somatic and psychiatric comorbidity in war veterans with post-traumatic stress disorder: preliminary findings. *Psychiatr Danub* 18:169–176.

Jin H, Lanouette NM, Mudaliar S, et al. 2009. Association of posttraumatic stress disorder with increased prevalence of metabolic syndrome. *J Clin Psychopharmacol.* 29:210–215.

Kang HK, Bullman TA, Taylor JW. 2006. Risk of selected cardiovascular diseases and posttraumatic stress disorder among former World War II prisoners of war. *Ann Epidemiol.* 16:381–386.

Kessler RC, McGonagle KA, Zhao S, et al. 1994. Lifetime and 12-month prevalence of DSM-III-R psychiatric disorders in the United States. *Arch Gen Psych.* 51:8–19.

Kibler JL. 2009. Posttraumatic stress and cardiovascular disease risk. *J Trauma Dissociation.* 10:135–150.

Kibler JL, Kavita J, Ma M. 2009. Hypertension in relation to posttraumatic stress disorder and depression in the US National Comorbidity Survey. *Behav Med.* 34:125–131.

Kimerling R. 2004. An investigation of sex differences in nonpsychiatric morbidity associated with posttraumatic stress disorder. *J Am Med Womens Assoc.* 59:43–47.

Kress AM, Hartzel MC, Peterson MR. 2005. Burden of disease associated with overweight and obesity among U.S. military retirees and their dependents, aged 38–64, 2003. *Prev Med.* 41:63–69.

Kress AM, Peterson MR, Hartzell MC. 2006. Association between obesity and depressive symptoms among U.S. Military active duty service personnel, 2002. *J Psychosomatic Res.* 60:263–271.

Kuo LE, Czarnecka M, Kitlinska JB, et al. 2008. Chronic stress, combined with a high-fat/high-sugar diet, shifts sympathetic signaling toward neuropeptide Y and leads to obesity and the metabolic syndrome. *Ann N Y Acad Sci.* 1148:232–237.

Lader M. 1974. The peripheral and central role of the catecholamines in the mechanisms of anxiety. *Int Pharmacopsychiatry.* 9:125–137.

Lauterbach D, Vora R, Rakow M. 2005. The relationship between posttraumatic stress disorder and self-reported health problems. *Psychosom Med.* 67:939–947.

Maes M, Lin AH, Delmeire L, et al. 1999. Elevated serum interleukin-6 (IL-6) and IL-6 receptor concentrations in posttraumatic stress disorder following accidental man-made traumatic events. *Biol Psychiatry.* 45:833–839.

Marmot M, Brunner E. 2005. Cohort profile: The Whitehall II study. *Int J Epidemiol.* 34:251–256.

Maslov B, Marcinko D, Millicevic R, et al. 2009. Metabolic syndrome, anxiety, depression and suicidal tendencies in post-traumatic stress disorder and schizophrenic patients. *Coll Antropol.* 33 Suppl 2:7–10.

McEwen BS, Stellar E. 1993. Stress and the individual. Mechanisms leading to disease. *Arch Intern Med.* 153:2093–2101.

McFarlane AC. 2010. The long-term costs of traumatic stress: intertwined physical and psychological consequences. *World Psychiatry.* 9:3–10.

Nelson KM. 2006. The burden of obesity among a national probability sample of veterans. *J Gen Intern Med.* 21:915–919.

Norman SB, Means-Christensen AJ, Craske MG, et al. 2006. Associations between psychological trauma and physical illness in primary care. *J Trauma Stress.* 19:461–470.

O'Toole BI, Catts SV. 2008. Trauma, PTSD, and physical health: an epidemiological study of Australian Vietnam veterans. *J Psychosom Res.* 64:33–40.

Rasmusson AM, Schnurr PP, Zukowska Z, et al. 2010. Adaptation to extreme stress: post-traumatic stress disorder, neuropeptide Y and metabolic syndrome. *Exp Biol Med (Maywood).* 235:1150–1162.

Reilly MP, Rader DJ. 2003. The metabolic syndrome: more than the sum of its parts? *Circulation.* 108:1546–1551.

Rohleder N, Karl A. 2006. Role of endocrine and inflammatory alterations in comorbid somatic diseases of post-traumatic stress disorder. *Minerva Endocrinol.* 31:273–288.

Schnurr PP, Ford JD, Friedman MJ, et al. 2000. Predictors and outcomes of posttraumatic stress disorder in World War II veterans exposed to mustard gas. *J Consult Clin Psychol.* 68:258–268.

Schnurr PP, Spiro A, Paris AH. 2000. Physician-diagnosed medical disorders in relation to PTSD symptoms in older male military veterans. *Health Psychol.* 19:91–97.

Spivak B, Shohat B, Mester R, et al. 1997. Elevated levels of serum interleukin-1 beta in combat-related posttraumatic stress disorder. *Biol Psychiatry.* 42:345–348.

Trief PM, Ouimette P, Wade M, et al. 2006. Post-traumatic stress disorder and diabetes: co-morbidity and outcomes in a male veterans sample. *J Behav Med.* 29:411–418.

Tucker P, Ruwe WD, Masters B, et al. 2004. Neuroimmune and cortisol changes in selective serotonin reuptake inhibitor and placebo treatment of chronic posttraumatic stress disorder. *Biol Psychiatry.* 56:121–128.

Vieweg WVR, Fernandez A, Julius DA, et al. 2006. Body mass index relates to males with posttraumatic stress disorder. *J Natl Med Assoc.* 98:580–586.

Vieweg WVR, Julius DA, Fernandez A, et al. 2006. Posttraumatic stress disorder in male military veterans with comorbid overweight and obesity: psychotropic, antihypertensive, and metabolic medications. *J Clin Psychiatry.* 8:25–31.

Vieweg WVR, Julius DA, Bates J, et al. 2007. Posttraumatic stress disorder as a risk factor for obesity among male military veterans. *Acta Psychiatr Scand.* 116:483–487.

Violante JM, Fekedulegn D, Hartley TA, et al. 2006. Police trauma and cardiovascular disease: association between PTSD symptoms and metabolic syndrome. *Int J Emerg Ment Health.* 8:227–237.

Wang A, Kinsinger LS, Kahwati LC, et al. 2005. Obesity and weight control practices in 2000 among veterans using VA facilities. *Obes Res.* 13:1405–1411.

Weisberg RB, Bruce SE, Machan JT, et al. 2002. Nonpsychiatric illness among primary care patients with trauma histories and posttraumatic stress disorder. *Psychiatr Serv.* 53:848–854.

Yarnell JWG, Patterson CC, Thomas HF, et al. 2000. Comparison of weight in middle age, weight at 18 years, and weight change between, in predicting subsequent 14 year mortality and coronary events: Caerphilly Prospective Study. *J Epidemiol Community Health.* 54:344–348.

Yehuda R, Boisoneau D, Mason JW, et al. 1993. Glucocorticoid receptor number and cortisol excretion in mood, anxiety, and psychotic disorders. *Biol Psychiatry.* 34:18–25.

7

Post-Traumatic Stress Disorder and Cardiovascular Disease

Steven S. Coughlin, Ph.D.

The topics dealt with in this chapter include studies of post-traumatic stress disorder (PTSD) as a predictor of cardiovascular disease. This includes possible biological mechanisms that may account for observed associations between PTSD and cardiovascular disease, and additional studies of PTSD occurring in the aftermath of potentially life-threatening events such as myocardial infarction, cardiac arrest, and stroke.

Major forms of cardiovascular disease include those attributed to atherosclerosis such as coronary heart disease and thromboembolic stroke. Coronary heart disease may develop as a result of hemodynamic factors (for example, elevated blood pressure with turbulence and sheer stress within coronary arteries), hyperlipidemia, and metabolic factors associated with the release of catecholamines (for example, platelet aggregation). Other events that may lead to myocardial infarction include the rupture of atherosclerotic plaques, thrombus formation, and vasospasm (Boscarino and Chang 1999).

Cardiovascular alterations associated with autonomic arousal and cardiovascular health outcomes have long been reported to be associated with PTSD or wartime traumatic exposures (Boscarino 2004; McFarlane 2010). Persons suffering from PTSD and chronic PTSD have been shown to have increases in basal heart rate and blood pressure and increased heart rate and blood pressure in response to stimuli such as loud sounds and visual slides that remind them of the trauma (Gerardi et al. 1994; Keane et al. 1998; Bedi and Arora 2007; Kleim et al. 2010). In clinical studies involving small samples of veterans, plasma norepinephrine and 24-hour urine norepinephrine levels have been reported to be elevated among veterans with PTSD as compared to those without PTSD (Mason et al. 1988). The increases in plasma norepinephrine are more pronounced when PTSD patients are exposed to trauma-related stimuli such as loud tones (Shalev 1992). Stress and anxiety have been associated with increased plasma and urinary norepinephrine, epinephrine, and their metabolites, which are peripheral measures of the noradrenergic system, in healthy adults (Lader 1974; Bedi and Arora 2007).

The effects of traumatic exposures or chronic stress on the hypothalamic-pituitary-adrenal (HPA) axis and the autonomic nervous system have been examined in clinical studies and in animal models. The results of these studies indicate that PTSD can result in important neurobiological and psychophysiological changes (McFarlane 2010). Physiological dysregulation of the HPA axis and altered autonomic function may contribute to increases in cardiovascular risk factors reported in persons with PTSD. Increased activity of the sympathoadrenal axis might contribute to cardiovascular disease through the effects of catecholamines on the heart, vasculature, and platelet function (Bedi and Arora 2007). Platelet function is altered by elevated levels of circulating catecholamines. Acting on alpha-2a receptors on platelet membranes, catecholamines lead to increased platelet aggregation and other changes in platelet function (Anfossi and Trovati 1996; Bedi and Arora 2007). Catecholamine-induced alterations of platelet activity have been hypothesized to be a link between chronic stress, increased sympathoadrenal activation, and cardiovascular disease (Anfossi and Trovati 1996; Vidovic et al. 2010).

Studies have shown that patients with PTSD have higher heart rates at rest and reduced heart rate variability, which is consistent with increased sympathetic activity (Cohen et al. 2000; Bedi and Arora 2007). The finding that baseline heart rate is higher among veterans suffering from PTSD than among those without PTSD is consistent with chronic hyperstimulation of the autonomic nervous system. Alternatively, the finding could be an artifact due to the research participants being anxious about the impending psychophysiological assessment (Blanchard 1990). The individuals who participated in the studies may have experienced anxiety because they were anticipating exposure to stimuli that would remind them of traumatic events (Bedi and Arora 2007). Mcfall et al. (1992) examined basal heart rates and systolic and diastolic blood pressure among veterans with and without PTSD over an extended period and did not find any significant differences between the two groups. However, in a separate study by Gerardi et al. (1994), which included 32 Vietnam veterans with combat-related PTSD and 26 Vietnam era veterans with no combat exposures, those with PTSD had significantly higher heart rate and systolic and diastolic blood pressure. Buckley and Kaloupek (2001) completed a meta-analysis of reported studies of basal heart rate and blood pressure among persons with and without PTSD. A total of 34 studies were included with a total sample size across studies of 2,670 subjects. Their results suggested that, on average, persons with PTSD have an elevated basal heart rate as compared with persons without PTSD or those who were not exposed to trauma (Buckley and Kaloupek 2001). The average difference in resting heart rate between persons with or without PTSD was five beats per minute. Their meta-analysis also suggested that PTSD is associated with blood pressure elevations (Buckley and Kaloupek 2001). Persons with PTSD have also been reported to be more likely to have hypertension, hyperlipidemia, obesity, and cardiovascular disease (McFarlane 2010).

STUDIES OF PTSD AND HYPERTENSION

PTSD was associated with an increased risk of hypertension in the National Comorbidity Survey and in an epidemiologic study of Vietnam veterans from Australia (O'Toole and Catts 2008; Kibler et al. 2009). Because elevated diastolic and systolic blood pressure are established risk factors for cardiovascular disease, the apparent link between PTSD and hypertension may partially account for reported associations between PTSD and heart disease (McFarlane 2010). Cohen et al. (2009) examined associations between PTSD and hypertension and other cardiovascular risk factors using national data from veterans of Operation Enduring Freedom and Operation Iraqi Freedom (OEF/OIF) who sought care at Department of Veterans Affairs (VA) health care facilities. The majority of the PTSD patients in their cross-sectional study had comorbid mental health diagnoses including depression (53%), other anxiety disorder (29%), substance abuse disorder (10%), and other psychiatric diagnoses (33%). Veterans with mental health diagnoses had a significantly higher frequency of hypertension and other cardiovascular disease risk factors (Cohen et al. 2009). For example, among 65,603 male OEF/OIF veterans who had PTSD with or without other mental health diagnoses, the adjusted odds ratio for the association between PTSD and hypertension was 2.88 (95% confidence interval 2.79–2.97) after controlling for age, race (white, black, Hispanic, or other), component type, rank, branch of service, and multiple deployments (Cohen et al. 2009). Among 6,964 female OEF/OIF veterans who had PTSD with or without other mental health diagnoses, the adjusted odds ratio for the association between PTSD and hypertension was 2.88 (95% confidence interval 2.79–2.97) after controlling for age, race/ethnicity (white, black, Hispanic, or other), component type, rank, branch of service, and multiple deployments (Cohen et al. 2009).

PTSD AND HYPERLIPIDEMIA

There is increasing evidence from clinical studies that PTSD may have effects on lipid metabolism (Kagan et al. 1999; Solter et al. 2002; Trief et al. 2006). Karlovic et al. (2004) examined total cholesterol, LDL and HDL cholesterol, and triglycerides in Croatian war veterans with PTSD and patients with major depression. Those with PTSD had higher levels of cholesterol and LDL cholesterol, and triglycerides, on average, and lower HDL cholesterol levels as compared with the patients with major depression. In the study by Cohen et al. (2009) of associations between PTSD and cardiovascular risk factors among OEF/OIF veterans who sought care at VA health care facilities, veterans with mental health diagnoses had a significantly higher frequency of dyslipidemia (Cohen et al. 2009). For example, among 65,603 male OEF/OIF veterans who had PTSD with or without other mental health diagnoses, the adjusted odds ratio for the association between PTSD and dyslipidemia was 2.70 (95% confidence interval 2.63–2.78) after controlling for age, race/ethnicity (white, black, Hispanic, or other), component type, rank, branch of service, and multiple deployments (Cohen et al. 2009). Among 6,964 female OEF/OIF veterans who had PTSD with or without other mental health diagnoses, the adjusted odds ratio for the association between PTSD and dyslipidemia was 2.68 (95% confidence interval 2.44–2.95) after controlling for age, race/ethnicity (white, black, Hispanic, or other), component type, rank, branch of service, and multiple deployments (Cohen et al. 2009). Elevated levels of total cholesterol and triglycerides have also been observed among Brazilian police officers with PTSD (Maia et al. 2008).

PTSD AND CIGARETTE SMOKING

Several studies have shown that persons with PTSD are more likely to smoke cigarettes than persons without PTSD (Shalev et al. 1990; Beckham et al. 1995, 1997; Fu et al. 2007). Chronic disease risk factors such as cigarette smoking, obesity, and physical inactivity may cluster among veterans with combat-related PTSD (Chwastiak et al. 2011). Persons suffering from PTSD may smoke as a coping strategy for dealing with traumatic memories, depression, or anxiety. In a sample of 124 Vietnam veterans with PTSD, Beckham et al. (1995) found that smokers had higher levels of PTSD symptoms, which is consistent with greater severity of PTSD contributing to smoking behavior. A systematic review conducted by Fu et al. (2007) identified 45 studies that reported data on PTSD and cigarette smoking. Smoking rates were high among clinical samples of PTSD patients (40–86%) and in nonclinical populations with PTSD (34–61%). Most of the studies reviewed by Fu et al. (2007) showed a positive association between PTSD and smoking, with odds ratios ranging between 2.0 and 4.5. Cigarette smoking is likely to interact with other cardiovascular risk factors (for example, hypertension, hyperlipidemia, and heavy alcohol consumption) to substantially increase cardiovascular risk.

STUDIES OF PTSD AS A PREDICTOR OF CORONARY HEART DISEASE MORBIDITY AND MORTALITY

Positive associations between PTSD and cardiovascular disease (particularly coronary heart disease) have been observed in a growing number of studies of veterans and civilians who were exposed to combat or other traumatic experiences, as summarized in Table 7.1. The focus of these studies is on PTSD as a predictor of cardiovascular disease. Another study, which has not specifically looked at PTSD, showed that persons exposed to traumatic stress resulting from civil war in Beirut, Lebanon, had a higher risk of cardiovascular disease mortality (Sibai et al. 2001). Additional studies, summarized later in this chapter, have examined PTSD occurring post-myocardial infarction, cardiac arrest, or other life-threatening cardiac event. Although some of the studies summarized in Table 7.1 relied upon self-reported information about cardiovascular disease or had other design limitations, an increasing number of studies have prospectively examined PTSD as a predictor of physician-diagnosed cardiovascular disease. Taken overall, these results from observa-

Table 7.1. Studies of PTSD and Cardiovascular Disease Among Veterans and Civilian Populations Exposed to Traumatic Experiences.

Study	Sample	Study Design	Results	Limitations	Other Information
Falger et al. 1992	Male World War II (WWII) Dutch Resistance veterans (n=147), aged 60-65 years, and age- and sex-matched controls with recent hospitalization for myocardial infarction (MI) (n=65) or surgery (n=79).	Clinical interviews of surviving veterans conducted more than 4 decades after the war had ended. PTSD was assessed using structured interviews based on the 3rd edition of the Diagnostic and Statistical Manual of Mental Disorders (DSM-III).	The Resistance veterans, especially those with PTSD, scored higher than the matched controls on angina pectoris, type A behavior, life stressors, and vital exhaustion. About 10% of the veterans reported having had an MI in the past 15 years. About 56% percent of the veterans were currently suffering from PTSD.	The use of controls with recent MI may have partly obscured associations with cardiovascular risk factors. History of MI was based on self-reported information.	Half of these Resistance veterans had been arrested and incarcerated in Nazi prisons and forced labor and death camps. All were exposed to extraordinary wartime trauma.
Boscarino 1997	National sample of male Vietnam veterans (n=1,399) who served in the U.S. Army.	In-person interviews conducted about 20 years post-combat exposure. Circulatory diseases were assessed retrospectively.	After controlling for age, race, region of birth, enlistment status, volunteer status, Army marital status, Army medical profile, smoking history, substance abuse, education, income, and other factors, lifetime PTSD status was associated with reported circulatory diseases (odds ratio [OR] = 1.62, $p = 0.007$) and other illnesses after military service. About 63% (n = 332) had a lifetime history of PTSD.	Use of self-reported information about disease history. The response rate was 65%.	

(continued on next page)

Table 7.1. (*continued*)

Study	Sample	Study Design	Results	Limitations	Other Information
Boscarino and Chang 1999	National sample of male U.S. Army veterans who served in theatre during the Vietnam war (n=2,490) or during the same era (n=1,972).	Medical examinations (conducted about 17 years after combat exposures for Vietnam theatre veterans). Psychiatric evaluations included the Diagnostic Interview Schedule based on DSM-III.	After controlling for age, place of service, illicit drug use, medication use, race, body mass index, alcohol use, cigarette smoking, and education, PTSD was associated with ECG findings including atrioventricular (AV) conduction defects (OR =2.81, 95% confidence interval [CI] 1.03-7.66, $p < 0.05$) and infarctions (OR=4.44, 95% CI 1.20-16.43, $p < 0.05$).	The overall participation rate was 60%. Soldiers who served in theatre may have had greater exposure to toxic chemicals.	The average age of first onset of PTSD was 21 years.
Boscarino 2006	National sample of male U.S. Army veterans (n=15,288) who served during the Vietnam War era.	Cohort mortality study with 16 years of follow-up following completion of a telephone survey (or about 30 years after their military service).	After controlling for race, Army volunteer status, Army entry age, Army discharge status, Army illicit drug abuse, age, and other factors, PTSD among Vietnam theatre veterans was associated with cardiovascular mortality (hazards ratio = 1.7, $p = 0.034$), all-cause mortality, cancer, and external causes of death.	Adjustment was made for pack-years of cigarette smoking only when looking at cancer mortality.	

(continued on next page)

Table 7.1. (continued)

Study	Sample	Study Design	Results	Limitations	Other Information
Boscarino 2008	National sample of male Vietnam veterans (n=4,328) who served in the U.S. Army. The men were < 65 years of age at follow-up.	Cohort mortality study.	PTSD was assessed using two measures including one based on the DSM-III. Having more PTSD symptoms was positively associated with early-age heart disease mortality.		
Dobie et al. 2004	Female veterans (n=1,259) who received care at the VA Puget Sound Health Care System between October 1996 and January 1998.	Cross-sectional postal survey.	Of the eligible women who completed the survey, 21% screened positive for current PTSD (PTSD Checklist-Civilian Version score $\geq$ 50). A statistically nonsignificant association was observed with MI or coronary artery disease (OR = 1.8, 95% CI 0.9–3.6).	Study limitations include the cross-sectional design and the reliance on self-reported information about medical conditions.	

(continued on next page)

Table 7.1. (continued)

Study	Sample	Study Design	Results	Limitations	Other Information
Kang et al. 2006	Former WWII prisoners of war (n=19,442) and non-POW controls (n=9,728).	Review of health care utilization data for 10 years (1991–2000) from VA and non-VA health-care providers.	After adjustment for age and race, former POWs with PTSD had statistically significant increased risks of CVD, including ischemic heart disease and hypertension, as compared with both non-POWS and POWs without PTSD. The magnitude of the increased risk of ischemic heart disease was modest, however.	POWs might be more likely than the study controls to be in VA medical treatment files.	
Schnurr et al. 2000	Male combat veterans of WWII and the Korean conflict (n=605). The average age at study entry was 43.9 years. The majority of the men (98%) were white.	Follow-up study. Medical examinations were performed periodically beginning in 1960. PTSD symptoms were assessed in 1990.	PTSD was assessed using the Mississippi Scale for Combat-Related PTSD. PTSD symptoms were positively associated with the onset of arterial disorders (hazard ratio $= 1.3$, 95% CI 1.2–1.5) after controlling for age, smoking, alcohol consumption, and body mass index. The hazard ratios for hypertensive and ischemic cardiovascular disease were not significantly different than one (no association).	PTSD was not measured at the beginning of the study but rather in 1990 after many of the outcomes had already occurred.	

(continued on next page)

Table 7.1. *(continued)*

Study	Sample	Study Design	Results	Limitations	Other Information
Kubzansky et al. 2007	Community-dwelling men (n=1,002) from the greater Boston, Massachusetts area who were aged 21–80 years in 1961. Most (>90%) of the men are veterans and most were white. Men with preexisting coronary heart disease or diabetes were excluded.	Prospective cohort study.	PTSD was assessed using the Mississippi Scale for Combat-Related PTSD. For each standard deviation increase in PTSD symptom level, the age-adjusted relative risk for non-fatal and fatal myocardial infarction combined was 1.3 (95% CI 1.05–1.5).		The data were from the VA Normative Aging Study.
Kubzansky et al. 2009	Community-dwelling women who participated in the Baltimore cohort of the Epidemiologic Catchment Area Study (n=1,059).	Prospective cohort study that assessed incident coronary heart disease over a 14-year period.	Past year trauma and associated PTSD symptoms were assessed using the National Institute of Mental Health (NIMH) Diagnostic Interview Schedule. Women with five or more symptoms of PTSD were over three times more likely to develop coronary heart disease than those with no symptoms (age-adjusted OR = 3.2, 95% CI 1.3–8.0). The association persisted after further adjustment was made for coronary risk factors and depression or trait anxiety.		

(continued on next page)

Table 7.1. (*continued*)

Study	Sample	Study Design	Results	Limitations	Other Information
Dirkzwager et al. 2007	Sample of adult survivors (n=896) of a fire disaster in Enschede, Netherlands that killed 23 persons and destroyed or damaged almost 1,500 houses.	Longitudinal design. Electronic medical records from family practitioners (1 year and 4 years post-disaster) were used for surveillance. Survey data were also collected at 3 weeks and 18 months post-disaster to assess PTSD and physical health.	The Self-Rating Scale for PTSD was used to assess the condition. After controlling for demographic factors, smoking, and pre-disaster physical health, PTSD was positively associated with risk of new vascular problems (OR = 1.9, 95% CI 1.04-3.6).		
Spitzer et al. 2009	Community-dwelling adults in Germany (n=3,171).	Cross-sectional survey.	PTSD was assessed using the Structured Clinical Interview for Diagnostic and Statistical Manual of Mental Disorders, 4th Edition (DSM-IV). After controlling for demographic factors, smoking, body mass index, blood pressure, depression, and alcohol use disorders, PTSD was positively associated with angina (OR = 2.4, 95% CI 1.3-4.5), heart failure (OR = 3.4, 95% CI 1.9-6.0), and peripheral arterial disease.	Study limitations include the cross-sectional design and the reliance on self-reported information about medical conditions.	

(continued on next page)

Table 7.1. (*continued*)

Study	Sample	Study Design	Results	Limitations	Other Information
Johnson et al. 2010	Male residents of four U.S. communities (n=5,347).	Population-based study of the prevalence of subclinical atherosclerosis (carotid intima thickness and carotid plaque) measured non-invasively at two study visits (1987–1989 and 1990–1992).	Compared to non-combat veterans, non-veterans and combat veterans had higher age-adjusted mean carotid intima thickness. Differences remained for combat veterans after adjustment for race, father's education, and age at service entry but not years of service. No differences in carotid plaque were noted.	PTSD was not assessed in this study.	The data were from the Atherosclerosis Risk in Communities (ARIC) Study.
Kunnas et al. 2011	667 Finnish WWII veterans who were alive at the age of 55 years and who resided in Tampere, an urban city in southern Finland.	Health survey conducted in 1980 with follow-up for mortality. Physical war injury was based on self-report at the time of the baseline examination.	A total of 140 deaths from coronary heart disease were identified. Men who had been wounded or injured in action were 1.7 times (95% CI 1.1–2.5) more likely to die from coronary heart disease than other men in this sample.	PTSD was not assessed in this study. The sample was limited to men.	

(continued on next page)

Table 7.1. (*continued*)

Study	Sample	Study Design	Results	Limitations	Other Information
Ahmadi et al. 2011	637 veterans with known coronary artery disease (12.2% women, mean ages 61 years).	Cross-sectional study involving non-invasive coronary artery calcium scans, combined with a cohort mortality study.	In persons with PTSD, coronary artery calcium scores were significantly higher than in those without PTSD (76.1% vs. 59%, $p = 0.001$). In multivariable linear regression analysis, PTSD was an independent predictor of the presence and extent of atherosclerotic coronary artery disease ($p < 0.01$). During a mean follow-up of 42 months, the overall death rate was higher among subjects with PTSD compared with the non-PTSD group (17.1% vs. 10.4%, $p = 0.003$).	The generalizability of the study findings is uncertain.	

tional research provide considerable evidence that persons with PTSD have a higher risk of coronary heart disease morbidity and mortality.

STUDIES OF PTSD AS A PREDICTOR OF CEREBRAL VASCULAR DISEASE

There is some evidence from epidemiologic studies of an association between PTSD and cerebrovascular disease. Brass and Page (1996) found that former World War II prisoners of war (POWs) had a statistically nonsignificant increased risk of stroke. Among the 475 former POWs, 12.7% (20 of 158) of those with PTSD had strokes, compared with 7.6% (24 of 317) without PTSD (relative risk = 1.7, 95% confidence interval 0.95– 2.9). In a cross-sectional survey of female veterans who received care at the VA Puget Sound Health Care System, Dobie et al. (2004) found an association between PTSD and self-reported history of stroke. About 5% (13 of 256) of the female veterans with PTSD reported a history of stroke as compared with 3% (28 of 905) of those without PTSD (age-adjusted odds ratio = 2.9, 95% confidence interval 1.4–6.0). A study of trauma and PTSD among 3,171 male and female adults living in the general population of a German community found that persons with a history of trauma had a higher odds of stroke (odds ratio = 1.2, 95% confidence interval 1.0–1.5), angina pectoris, and heart failure after adjustment for demographic factors, blood pressure, smoking, body mass index, depression, and alcohol-related disorders (Spitzer et al. 2009).

STUDIES OF PTSD OCCURRING POST-MYOCARDIAL INFARCTION OR OTHER POTENTIALLY LIFE-THREATENING CARDIOVASCULAR EVENT

Myocardial infarction is a stressful, potentially life-threatening medical emergency which can lead to serious complications, recurrent cardiac events, or death. The stress of experiencing a myocardial infarction is intensified by the suddenness of the event and the general lack of control by the victim (Ginzburg et al. 2002). An estimated 10–20% of patients develop PTSD as a consequence of the traumatic experience of suffering a myocardial infarction (Gander and Von Kanel 2006; von Kanel et al. 2011). PTSD can be diagnosed, at the earliest, one month following a myocardial infarction or other traumatic event. A review of the literature on PTSD post-myocardial infarction noted the wide variety of study designs, sampling procedures, and approaches used to assess PTSD (Spindler and Pedersen 2005). For example, many studies have not used structured clinical interviews to assess PTSD. Nevertheless, several important findings have been reported in studies conducted to date. Follow-up studies of post-myocardial infarction patients have identified predictors of post-traumatic stress including intense pain and feelings of helplessness at the time of the myocardial infarction, subjective perception of threat to life, anticipated incapacitation after the myocardial infarction, lack of social support, prior traumatization, younger age, and female sex (Spindler and Pedersen 2005; Rocha et al. 2008; Guler et al. 2009; Hari et al. 2010; Roberge et al. 2010), although female sex and pain intensity were not found to be predictive of PTSD in some studies of post-myocardial infarction patients (Wiedemar et al. 2008; Roberge et al. 2010). Myocardial infarction patients often experience major depression, which can co-occur with PTSD and other anxiety disorders in these patients (Shemesh et al. 2006).

Follow-up studies have shown that post-myocardial infarction patients who develop PTSD may be less likely to adhere to treatment recommendations such as taking prescription medications or aspirin, than patients without PTSD, and that they may be more likely to be readmitted to a hospital for a cardiovascular condition (Shemesh et al. 2001, 2004), although PTSD was not associated with poorer medication adherence in one study of post-myocardial infarction patients (Jones et al. 2007). It is possible that myocardial infarction survivors with PTSD view medical recommendations as traumatic reminders (Shemesh et al. 2006). PTSD may worsen medical outcomes among post-myocardial infarction patients by increasing non-adherence to medication regimens (Shemesh 2004).

Post-myocardial infarction patients who undergo bypass surgery or angioplasty and cardiac arrest survivors may also be more likely to develop PTSD (O'Reilly et al. 2004; Chung et al. 2008). Patients who undergo cardiac surgery, cardiac transplantation, or who suffer acute pulmonary failure, an acute exacerbation of congestive heart failure, edema, or a stroke (including subarachnoid haemorrhage) may also have an increased risk of developing PTSD (Tedstone and Tarrier 2003; Cotter et al. 2006; Sheldrick et al. 2006; Schelling 2008), although more research is needed to confirm and clarify these findings. Patients who are treated in an intensive care unit with mechanical ventilation have also been reported to have an increased risk of PTSD (Weinert 2005; Schelling 2008).

SUMMARY AND CONCLUSIONS

This review of the published literature highlights evidence from epidemiologic and clinical studies that persons with PTSD are at increased risk of cardiovascular disease including coronary heart disease and possibly stroke. The biological mechanisms that may account for the observed associations may relate to the effects of traumatic exposures and chronic stress on the HPA axis and the autonomic nervous system (Bedi and Arora 2007). Dysregulation of the HPA axis and chronic overstimulation of the autonomic nervous system may contribute to the increases in blood pressure and lipid levels that have been observed in PTSD patients. In addition, persons with PTSD are more likely to be heavy alcohol drinkers or cigarette smokers, which are known risk factors for hypertension and heart disease. Catecholamine-induced alterations of platelet activity may also contribute to the apparent link between PTSD and cardiovascular disease. Changes in immune function seen in some PTSD patients may also have a role including circulating levels of interleukin-6 (IL-6), IL-1, tumor necrosis factor, and C-reactive protein (Rohleder and Karl 2006). Inflammatory mediators such as IL-6, tumor necrosis factor, and C-reactive protein have been reported to stimulate atherosclerosis (Rohleder and Karl 2006). Interactions among the immune and neuroendocrine systems may partly account for associations between PTSD and chronic disease outcomes.

Previous authors have proposed general models of possible mechanisms underlying the relationship between PTSD and physical health including cardiovascular disease (Schnurr and Jankowski 1999; Schnurr and Green 2004). The models take into account biological function (e.g., HPA axis, heightened noradrenergic function, immune function), psychological comorbidities such as depression, health risk behaviors, symptom reports and functional status, and disease morbidity and mortality. A similar model of PTSD outcomes proposed by Boscarino (2004) accounts for different pathways leading to changes in health status; the influences of heredity, shared environment, history of trauma, behavior and perceptions, biological changes, and stressful life event exposures are taken into account in the model.

Given the evidence from clinical research that persons who survive a myocardial infarction (or other life-threatening and extremely stressful cardiac, cerebrovascular, or pulmonary event) have an increased risk of PTSD (Spindler and Pedersen 2005; Shemesh et al. 2006; Roberge et al. 2010; von Kanel et al. 2011), the relationship between PTSD and cardiovascular disease is one of dual causation. PTSD is both a predictor of myocardial infarction and other cardiovascular conditions and a potential adverse outcome among myocardial infarction survivors. Previously proposed models of mechanisms or pathways that account for associations between PTSD and physical health outcomes (Schnurr and Jankowski 1999; Boscarino 2004; Schnurr and Green 2004) can be extended and enhanced to take into account the complex natural history of PTSD and associated chronic health conditions such as myocardial infarction. Such models should ideally highlight opportunities for primary, secondary, and tertiary prevention. The latter is an increasingly important part of cardiovascular death reduction, as the number of persons who survive a myocardial infarction has increased due to improvements in medical and surgical treatment and because of the aging of the population (Spindler and Pedersen 2005).

REFERENCES

Ahmadi N, Hajsadeghi F, Mirshkario HB, et al. 2011. Post-traumatic stress disorder, coronary atherosclerosis, and mortality. *Am J Cardiol.* 108:29–33.

Anfossi G, Trovati M. 1996. Role of catecholamines in platelet function: pathophysiological and clinical significance. *Eur J Clin Invest.* 26:353–370.

Beckham JC, Roodman AA, Shipley RH, et al. 1995. Smoking in Vietnam combat veterans with post-traumatic stress disorder. *J Trauma Stress.* 8:461–472.

Beckham JC, Kirby AC, Feldman ME, et al. 1997. Prevalence and correlates of heavy smoking in Vietnam veterans with chronic posttraumatic stress disorder. *Addictive Behav.* 22:637–647.

Bedi US, Arora R. 2007. Cardiovascular manifestations of posttraumatic stress disorder. *J National Med Assoc.* 99:642–649.

Blanchard EB. 1990. Elevated basal levels of cardiovascular responses in Vietnam veterans with PTSD: a health problem in the making? *J Anxiety Disord.* 4:233–237.

Boscarino JA. 1997. Diseases among men 20 years after exposure to severe stress: implications for clinical research and medical care. *Psychosomatic Med.* 59:605–614.

Boscarino JA. 2004. Posttraumatic stress disorder and physical illness. Results from clinical and epidemiologic studies. *Ann NY Acad Sci.* 1032:141–153.

Boscarino JA. 2008. A prospective study of PTSD and early-age heart disease mortality among Vietnam veterans: implications for surveillance and prevention. *Psychosomatic Med.* 70:668–676.

Boscarino JA, Chang J. 1999. Electrocardiogram abnormalities among men with stress-related psychiatric disorders: implications for coronary heart disease and clinical research. *Ann Behavioral Med.* 21:227–234.

Brass LM, Page WF. 1996. Stroke in former prisoners of war. *J Stroke Cerebrovasc Dis.* 6:72–78.

Buckley TC, Kaloupek DG. 2001. A meta-analytic examination of basal cardiovascular activity in posttraumatic stress disorder. *Psychosomatic Med.* 63:585–594.

Chung MC, Berger Z, Rudd H. 2008. Coping with posttraumatic stress disorder and comorbidity after myocardial infarction. *Compr Psychiatry.* 49:55–64.

Chwastiak LA, Rosenheck RA, Desai R, Kazis LE. 2010. Association of psychiatric illness and all-cause mortlity in the National Department of Veterans Affairs Health Care System. *Psychosomatic Med.* 72:817–822.

Chwastiak LA, Rosenheck RA, Kazis LE. 2011. Association of psychiatric illness and obesity, physical inactivity, and smoking among a national sample of veterans. *Psychosomatics.* 52:230–236.

Cohen BE, Marmar C, Ren L, et al. 2009. Association of cardiovascular risk factors with mental health diagnoses in Iraq and Afghanistan war veterans using VA health care. *JAMA.* 302:489–492.

Cohen H, Benjamin J, Geva AB, et al. 2000. Autonomic dysregulation in panic disorder and in post-traumatic stress disorder: application of power spectrum analysis of heart rate variability at rest and in response to recollection of trauma or panic attacks. *Psychiatry Res.* 96:1–13.

Cotter G, Milo-Cotter O, Rubinstein D, Shemesh E. 2006. Posttraumatic stress disorder: a missed link between psychiatric and cardiovascular morbidity? *CNS Spectr.* 11:129–136.

Dobie DJ, Kivlahan DR, Maynard C, et al. 2004. Postraumatic stress disorder in female veterans. Association with self-reported health problems and functional impairment. *Arch Intern Med.* 164:394–400.

Fu S, McFall M, Saxon AJ, et al. 2007. Posttraumatic stress disorder and smoking: a systematic review. *Nicotine Tob Res.* 9:1071–1084.

Gander ML, von Kanel R. 2006. Myocardial infarction and post-traumatic stress disorder: frequency, outcome, and atherosclerotic mechanisms. *Eur J Cardiovasc Prev Rehabil.* 13:165–172.

Gerardi RJ, Keane TM, Cahoon BJ, Klauminzer GW. 1994. An in vivo assessment of physiological arousal in posttraumatic stress disorder. *J Abn Psychol.* 103:825–827.

Ginzburg K, Solomon Z, Bleich A. 2002. Repressive coping style, acute stress disorder, and posttraumatic stress disorder after myocardial infarction. *Psychosomatic Med.* 64:748–757.

Greenberg JB, Ameringer KJ, Trujillo MA, et al. 2011. Associations between posttraumatic stress disorder symptom clusters and cigarette smoking. *Psychol Addict Behav.* In press.

Guler E, Schmid JP, Wiedemar L, et al. 2009. Clinical diagnosis of posttraumatic stress disorder after myocardial infarction. *Clin Cardiol.* 32:125–129.

Hari R, Begre S, Schmid JP, et al. 2010. Change over time in posttraumatic stress caused by myocardial infarction and predicting variables. *J Psychosom Res.* 69:143–150.

Jones RCM, Chung MC, Berger Z, Campbell JL. 2007. Prevalence of post-traumatic stress disorder in patients with previous myocardial infarction consulting in general practice. *Br J Gen Practice.* 57:808–810.

Kagan BL, Leskin G, Haas B, et al. 1999. Elevated lipid levels in Vietnam veterans with chronic posttraumatic stress disorder. *Biol Psychiatry.* 45:374–7.

Kang HK, Bullman TA, Taylor JW. 2006. Risk of selected cardiovascular diseases and posttraumatic stress disorder among former World War II prisoners of war. *Ann Epidemiol.* 16:381–386.

Karlovic D, Buljan D, Martinac M, et al. 2004. Serum lipid concentrations in Croatian veterans with post-traumatic stress disorder, post-traumatic stress disorder comorbid with major depressive disorder, or major depressive disorder. *J Korean Med Sci.* 19:431–436.

Keane TM, Kolb LC, Kaloupek DG, et al. 1998. Utility of psychophysiological measurement in the diagnosis of posttraumatic stress disorder: results from a Department of Veterans Affairs cooperative study. *J Consult Clin Psychol.* 66:914–923.

Kibler JL, Joshi K, Ma M. 2009. Hypertension in relation to posttraumatic stress disorder and depression in the US National Comorbidity Survey. *Behav Med.* 34:125–132.

Kleim B, Wilhelm FH, Glucksman E, Ehlers A. 2010. Sex differences in heart rate responses to script-driven imagery soon after trauma and risk of posttraumatic stress disorder. *Psychosomatic Med.* 72:917–924.

Kubzansky LD, Koenen KC, Spiro A III, et al. 2007. Prospective study of posttraumatic stress disorder symptoms and coronary heart disease in the Normative Aging Study. *Arch Gen Psychiatry.* 64:109–116.

Kunnas T, Solakivi T, Renko J, et al. 2011. Late-life coronary heart disease mortality of Finnish war veterans in the TAMRISK study, a 28-year follow-up. *BMC Public Health.* 11:71.

Lader M. 1974. The peripheral and central role of the catecholamines in the mechanisms of anxiety. *Int Pharmacopsychiatry.* 9:125–137.

Maia DB, Marmar CR, Mendlowicz MV, et al. 2008. Abnormal serum lipid profile in Brazilian police officers with post-traumatic stress disorder. *J Affect Disord.* 107:259–263.

Mason JW, Giller EL, Kosten TR, Harkness L. 1988. Elevation of urinary norepinephrine/cortisol ratio in posttraumatic stress disorder. *J Nerv Mental Dis.* 176:498–502.

McFall ME, Veith RC, Murburg MM. 1992. Basal sympathoadrenal function in posttraumatic stress disorder. *Biol Psychiatry.* 31:1050–1056.

McFarlane AC. 2010. The long-term costs of traumatic stress: intertwined physical and psychological consequences. *World Psychiatry.* 9:3–10.

O'Reilly SM, Grubb N, O'Carroll RE. 2004. Long-term emotional consequences of in-hospital cardiac arrest and myocardial infarction. *Br J Clin Psychol.* 43(Part 1):83–95.

O'Toole BI, Catts SV. 2008. Trauma, PTSD, and physical health: an epidemiological study of Australian Vietnam veterans. *J Psychosom Res.* 64:33–40.

Perry BD, Giller EJ, Southwick SM. 1987. Altered platelet alpha-2 adrenergic binding sites in posttraumatic stress disorder (letter). *Am J Psychiatry.* 144:1324–1327.

Qureshi SU, Pyne JM, Magruder KM, et al. 2009. The link between post-traumatic stress disorder and physical comorbidities: a systematic review. *Psychiatr Q.* 80:87–97.

Roberge MA, Dupuis G, Marchand A. 2010. Post-traumatic stress disorder following myocardial infarction: prevalence and risk factors. *Can J Cardiol.* 26:e170–e175.

Rocha LP, Peterson JC, Meyers B, et al. 2008. Incidence of posttraumatic stress disorder (PTSD) after myocardial infarction (MI) and predictors of PTSD symptoms post-MI—a brief report. *Int J Psychiatry Med.* 38:297–306.

Rohleder N, Karl A. 2006. Role of endocrine and inflammatory alterations in comorbid somatic diseases of post-traumatic stress disorder. *Minerva Endocrinologica.* 31:273–288.

Schelling G. 2008. Post-traumatic stress disorder in somatic disease: lessons from critically ill patients. *Prog Brain Res.* 167:229–237.

Schnurr PP, Green BL. 2004. Understanding relationships among trauma, post-traumatic stress disorder, and health outcomes. *Advances Spring.* 20:18–29.

Shalev A, Bleich A, Ursano RJ. 1990. Posttraumatic stress disorder: somatic comorbidity and effort tolerance. *Psychosomatics.* 31:197–203.

Shalev AY, Orr SP, Peri T, et al. 1992. Physiologic responses to loud tones in Israeli patients with posttraumatic stress disorder. *Arch Gen Psychiatry.* 49:870–874.

Sheldrick R, Tarrier N, Berry E, Kincey J. 2006. Post-traumatic stress disorder and illness perceptions over time following myocardial infarction and subarachnoid haemorrhage. *Bri J Health Psychol.* 11(Part 3):387–400.

Shemesh E, Koren-Michowitz M, Yehuda R, et al. 2006. Symptoms of posttraumatic stress disorder in patients who have had a myocardial infarction. *Psychosomatics.* 47:231–239.

Shemesh E, Rudnick A, Kaluski E, et al. 2001. A prospective study of posttraumatic stress symptoms and nonadherence in survivors of a myocardial infarction (MI). *Gen Hosp Psychiatry.* 23:215–222.

Shemesh E, Yehuda R, Milo O, et al. 2004. Posttraumatic stress, nonadherence, and adverse outcome in survivors of a myocardial infarction. *Psychosomatic Med.* 66:521–526.

Sibai AM, Fletcher AF, Armenian HK. 2001. Variations in the impact of long-term wartime stressors on mortality among the middle-aged and older population in Beirut, Lebanon, 1983–1993. *Am J Epidemiol.* 154:128–137.

Solter V, Thaller V, Karlovic D, et al. 2002. Elevated serum lipids in veterans with combat-related chronic posttraumatic stress disorder. *Croat Med J.* 43:685–689.

Spindler H, Pedersen SS. 2005. Posttraumatic stress disorder in the wake of heart disease: prevalence, risk factors, and future research directions. *Psychosomatic Med.* 67:715–723.

Spitzer C, Barnow S, Volzke H, et al. 2009. Trauma, posttraumatic stress disorder, and physical illness: findings from the general population. *Psychosom Med.* 71:1012–1017.

Tedstone JE, Tarrier N. 2003. Posttraumatic stress disorder following medical illness and treatment. *Clin Psychol Rev.* 23:409–448.

Trief PM, Ouimette P, Wade M, et al. 2006. Post-traumatic stress disorder and diabetes: co-morbidity and outcomes in a male veterans sample. *J Behav Med.* 29:411–418.

Vidovic A, Grubisic-llic M, Kozaric-Kovacic D, et al. 2010. Exaggerated platelet reactivity to physiological agonists in war veterans with posttraumatic stress disorder. *Psychoneuroendocrinology.* 36:161–172.

von Kanel R, Hari R, Schmid JP, et al. 2011. Non-fatal cardiovascular outcome in patients with posttraumatic stress symptoms caused by myocardial infarction. *J Cardiol* 58:61–68.

von Kanel R, Mills PJ, Fainman C, Dimsdale JE. 2001. Effects of psychological stress and psychiatric disorders on blood coagulation and fibrinolysis: a biobehavioral pathway to coronary artery disease? *Psychosomatic Med.* 63:531–544.

Weinert C. 2005. Epidemiology and treatment of psychiatric conditions that develop after critical illness. *Curr Opin Crit Care.* 11:376–380.

Wiedemar L, Schmid JP, Muller J, et al. 2008. Prevalence and predictors of posttraumatic stress disorder in patients with acute myocardial infarction. *Heart Lung.* 37:113–121.

8

Post-Traumatic Stress Disorder and Traumatic Brain Injury

Steven S. Coughlin, Ph.D., Patrick M. Sullivan, M.A., and
Julie C. Chapman, Psy.D.

Traumatic brain injuries (TBI) result from the transfer of mechanical energy to the brain from external forces and are exacerbated by secondary biochemical cascades in the hours and days following the primary or "mechanical" injury. In the immediate aftermath of the primary injury, TBI is manifested by disorientation or frank loss of consciousness (LOC), post-traumatic amnesia (PTA), or other neurologic symptoms. These manifestations, combined with brain imaging results and Glasgow Coma Score (Teasdale and Jennett 1974), if available, are used to classify the injury as mild, moderate, or severe for the purposes of clinical diagnosis and prognosis. The phrase "natural recovery period" refers to the general time periods associated with the body's inherent healing processes and varies with the severity of the injury. These estimates provide rough guidelines that are impacted by poorly understood factors specific to the individual patient.

Following a concussion or mild TBI (mTBI), common symptoms include dizziness, problems with balance/equilibrium, headaches, ringing in the ears, sleep problems, and irritability or mood disturbance. Cognitive problems in the domains of attention, memory, and executive dysfunction are also reported. The latter include higher-level cognitive operations, such as planning, initiating, organizing, mental flexibility, insight, and judgment that are heavily dependent upon the prefrontal cortex of the brain (McCullagh and Feinstein 2011). Among individuals sustaining an mTBI, up to 24% continue to have significant impairment at three months post-injury according to Ponsford et al. (Ponsford et al. 2000). This prevalence rate is supported by a recent two-site study (Faux et al. 2011) which showed prevalence rates of 25.6% and 35.1% for post-concussive disorder at three months post-injury.

Moderate TBI (ModTBI) has been associated with a wide array of neuropsychiatric symptoms, some of which are similar, but inherently more serious than those found in mTBI, and others that differ. In addition to greater difficulties with attention, memory, and executive functioning, ModTBI patients may also exhibit more focal neurocognitive deficits, such as problems with language (i.e., anomia, aphasia) and visuospatial processing. Sensory perception and reception may also be disrupted (e.g., smell, vision, hearing, touch, and taste). Physiological symptoms such as headache, chronic pain, and disequilibrium/proprioception are frequently present (Department of Veterans Affairs [VA] 2010). Finally, greater neurobehavioral disturbances are seen (i.e., mood, anxiety, agitation, sleep problems, loss of libido) than are observed in patients sustaining a mTBI. In addition to more serious manifestations of the above symptoms, *sequela* of severe TBI can include minimally conscious states, coma or death. The natural recovery period for moderate to severe TBI is variable (Hellawell 1999) and typically results in life-long physical, cognitive, social, and emotional consequences (Langlois et al. 2006). A comparison of TBI and post-traumatic stress disorder (PTSD) symptomatology are summarized later in this chapter.

RATES OF TBI IN CIVILIAN, MILITARY, AND VETERAN POPULATIONS

The Centers for Disease Control and Prevention (CDC) estimated the annual U.S. incidence of TBI at 1.7 million (Faul et al. 2010). However, it is likely that CDC rates underestimate the incidence of TBI due to the suspected large number of unreported brain injuries each year. Additionally, CDC rates do not include combat-related injuries as reported by the U.S. Department of Defense (DoD) and the Veterans Health Administration. Groups at increased risk for TBI include persons who participate in contact sports such as football and boxing; civilians who are injured as the result of motor vehicle accidents, falls, other types of accidents (for example, colliding with a moving or stationary object), or who are the victims of assault/interpersonal violence; and military troops exposed to combat (Collins et al. 2002; Guskiewicz et al. 2003; Terrio et al. 2009; DeKosy et al. 2010; Faul et al. 2010).

The increased incidence of blast-related TBI in Afghanistan, Operation Enduring Freedom (OEF), and Iraq, Operation Iraqi Freedom (OIF) and Operation New Dawn (OND), in recent years can be attributed to several factors. The use of high-order explosives by insurgent groups, particularly in the form of improvised explosive devises, has armed the enemy in new and dangerous ways. However, the defining and salient contributors to the increased incidence of TBI relate to the prevention of death that has been associated with TBI in prior conflicts. Innovations in protective gear for U.S. military personnel and improvements in medical and surgical care for traumatic injuries (Warden 2005, 2006) have led to the survival of injuries that would have resulted in certain death just decades prior.

Precise estimates of the prevalence of TBI in OEF/OIF/OND veterans are currently lacking. About three-quarters of all types of combat injuries in OEF/OIF have been the results of explosive munitions (Owens et al. 2008). Several groups (Vasterling et al. 2006; Schwab et al. 2007; Galarneau et al. 2008; Hoge et al. 2008; Schell and Marshall 2008; Schneiderman et al. 2008; Terrio et al. 2009) have estimated the prevalence of TBI among military personnel and veterans who were deployed to OEF/OIF. These estimates have ranged from 8% to 23%. The wide range is likely due to differences in sample definition and TBI evaluation method (e.g., self-reported information from a population survey, in-person interview and evaluation by a health care professional, etc.). Vasterling et al. (2006) reported the rate of TBI among OEF/OIF veterans as 7.6%. However, TBI was defined to require a loss of consciousness of 15 minutes or longer. As the diagnostic criteria for mTBI do not require a loss of consciousness and given that mTBI comprises the largest percentage of all severities, this result is likely a significant underestimate.

From a survey of 2,525 service members from two infantry brigades, Hoge et al. (2008) reported a 15% prevalence rate of TBI among the OEF/OIF cohort. Although the sample size was large, the determination of the TBI diagnosis was based upon self-reported measures with no clinician involvement. Additionally, these service members reported PTSD symptoms. Using multivariate logistical regression analysis, Hoge et al. (2008) observed that the relationship between loss of consciousness and TBI symptoms was mediated by PTSD and depression. However, given that multiple groups have shown microstructural change as a result of mTBI (Kraus 2007; Rutgers et al. 2008; Wilde et al. 2008; Niogi 2010; MacDonald et al. 2011), further research is needed to clarify this relationship.

RAND Corporation (Tanielian and Jaycox 2008) conducted a large (n = 1,938), geographically representative survey of health conditions following deployment to OEF/OIF. Data collected by clinicians conducting telephone surveys using validated instruments yielded prevalence estimates as high as 23% and 17% for TBI and PTSD, respectively. Midpoint estimates were 19.5% for TBI and 13.8% for PTSD. These estimates provide one of the most reliable indications of the prevalence of these two conditions in OEF/OIF veterans at the current time. Although TBI and PTSD frequently co-occur in clinical practice, Tanielian and Jaycox (2008) found only a small estimated overlap of 1.1%.

In addition to results from these peer-reviewed studies, media reports have provided additional information about the frequency of TBI among selected military populations. For example, according to a 2006 report in USA Today, 10% of 7,909 Marines with the 1st Marine Division at Camp Pendleton, California, suffered brain injuries (Zoroya 2006). At Fort Irwin in California, 1,490 soldiers who had served in combat were screened, and close to 12% suffered concussions during deployment (Zoroya 2006).

MECHANISMS OF BLAST INJURIES

Brain injury as a result of blast is defined by the types of blast mechanisms, which are categorized as primary, secondary, tertiary, or quaternary. The primary mechanism of blast-related TBI occurs as a result of the blast wave, which creates rapid changes in the atmospheric pressure (Terrio et al. 2009). Blast was defined by Moore and Jaffee (2010) as "an explosion in the atmosphere characterized by the release of energy in such a short period of time and within such a small volume resulting in the creation of a non-linear shock and pressure wave of finite amplitude, spreading from the source of detonation." Secondary and tertiary mechanisms of blast injury refer to the head being struck by flying debris and to body displacement, respectively. Quaternary mechanisms of blast (injuries due to additional features associated with exposure to high-order explosions) include inhalation of toxic fumes, burns, and crush injuries (Belanger et al. 2009).

Blast injuries can lead to rupture of the tympanic membrane and temporary deafness, tinnitus, and vertigo due to neurapraxia in the receptor organs of the ear (DePalma et al. 2005). In mass casualty situations, auditory system injuries and concussions are easily overlooked because the symptoms of mTBI are so similar to the symptoms of PTSD (CDC 2003).

Accurate screening, diagnosis and treatment of blast-related mTBI and combat-related PTSD may be greatly facilitated by illumination of the underlying pathophysiology of each. The pathogenesis of blast-related brain injury is the subject of current study and debate (Hicks et al. 2010). Cernak and Noble-Haeusslein (2010) reported two hypothesized pathways of blast energy transmission to the brain: (1) direct transcranial dissemination, where the blast wave moves through the skull into the brain (Bhattacharjee 2008); and (2) peripheral vascular propagation (the large vessels in the body transmit blast energy to the central nervous system via the vasculature; Courtney and Courtney 2009). The physics underlying blast-related brain injury in the context of current conflicts are multifaceted (Cernak and Noble-Haeusslein 2010), non-linear (Moore and Jaffee 2010), and consequently difficult to model. Additional meticulous research must be done before firm conclusions can be drawn.

As is true in civilian populations, the majority of brain injuries occurring among combat troops are mild in severity and often do not require hospitalization (Terrio 2009). However, combat troops may also suffer from moderate or severe brain injury, resulting in polytrauma or multiple complex injuries involving more than one physical region or organ system (Belanger et al. 2009).

SCREENING AND DIAGNOSIS OF TBI HIGHER-RISK GROUPS

Current diagnostic procedures for TBI in both military and civilian populations rely heavily on patient self-report, which is an important source of information in diagnosis. However, TBI can impact an individual's ability to recall or to communicate important aspects of the event. The identification of objective measures may improve the speed of screening and accuracy of diagnosis. As such, there is currently no "gold standard" for screening patients for TBI. However, ongoing studies are attempting to validate assessment tools by comparing resulting data with information gained from magnetic resonance imaging (MRI) and other noninvasive imaging technologies. A study by Chapman et al. (2010) demonstrated that a neurologic battery, the Brief Objective Neurobehavioral Detector was able to distinguish mTBI from comorbid psychiatric conditions with high degrees of sensitivity and specificity. Other studies, such as the experimental test for proteins in the blood that was announced in 2010 by the DoD and a Florida biotechnology company, are examining biomarkers of traumatic brain injury. Ongoing research by Chapman et al. (2010) is investigating the use of a multimodal diagnosis model for blast-related mTBI. Cognitive, neurological, and multiple imaging modalities are being used to develop enduring biomarkers for mTBI. This study will serve as the launching platform for the Markers for the Identification, Norming, and Differentiation of TBI and PTSD Study, a multicenter study aimed at a comprehensive, multidisciplinary description of mTBI and PTSD.

In order to screen troops returning from deployment in Afghanistan and Iraq, the U.S. Army and the Department of Veterans Affairs have developed screening tools for traumatic brain injury (Belanger et al. 2009; Schwab et al. 2009; Terrio et al. 2009, 2011). The DoD has included questions pertaining to traumatic brain injury in the Post Deployment Health Assessment form completed for troops returning from deployment. Screening tools for traumatic brain injury may be especially useful for identifying milder injuries that are less obvious and which result in no loss of consciousness or only short periods of unconsciousness (Schwab et al. 2007).

The Brief Traumatic Brain Injury Screen (BTBIS) is a one-page paper-and-pencil questionnaire designed to screen soldiers for traumatic brain injury. This screening tool allows individuals to self-report probable traumatic brain injury and symptoms that are associated with the condition, so that they may be triaged for further evaluation, diagnosis, and treatment. Respondents are asked:

Did you have any injury(ies) during your deployment from any of the following? (check all that apply): (1) Fragment; (2) Bullet; (3) Vehicular (any type of vehicle, including airplane); (4) Fall; (5) Explosion (improvised explosive device, rocket propelled grenade, land mine, grenade, etc.); (6) Other (specify).

In addition, they are asked:

Did any injury you received while deployed result in any of the following? (check all that apply): (1) Being dazed, confused, or "seeing stars"; (2) Not remembering the injury; (3) Losing consciousness (knocked out) for less than a minute; (4) Losing consciousness for 1–20 minutes; (5) Losing consciousness for longer than 20 minutes; (6) Having any symptoms of concussion afterward (such as headache, dizziness, irritability, etc.); (7) Head injury; (8) None of the above.

Lastly, respondents are asked:

Are you currently experiencing any of the following problems that you think might be related to a possible head injury or concussion (check all that apply): (1) Headaches; (2) Dizziness; (3) Memory problems; (4) Balance problems; (5) Ringing in the ears; (6) Irritability; (7) Sleep problems; (8) Other (specify).

The BTBIS was designed without reference to head injury or traumatic brain injury so as to encourage a wide self-report of possible traumatic brain injury (Schwab et al. 2007). Although studies of its reliability and validity are needed, preliminary assessment of the usefulness of BTBIS as a screening tool for traumatic brain injury suggested that it could be useful to triage persons in mass casualty situations such as persons returning from combat (Schwab et al. 2007).

The Department of Veterans Affairs uses a four-question screening tool for traumatic brain injury which is a modified version of the BTBIS (Belanger et al. 2009). The screening tool is part of a series of clinical reminders for OEF/OIF/OND veterans seen at Department of Veterans Affairs (VA) health care facilities. The traumatic brain injury clinical reminder was incorporated into the VA computerized medical record system in 2007 (Belanger et al. 2009). If the veteran has not already been identified as having a traumatic brain injury, they are asked the following questions:

(1) Did you have any injury(ies) during your deployment from any of the following?" (check all that apply: fragment, bullet, explosion, etc.); (2) Did any injury you received while deployed result in any of the following (check all that apply: being dazed, confused or "seeing stars," not remembering the injury, losing consciousness, head injury, etc.); (3) Did any of these begin or

get worse afterward (check all that apply: dizziness, headaches, memory problems, balance problems, ringing in the ears, irritability, sleep problems); and (4) In the past week, have you had any of the above symptoms (check all that apply: dizziness, memory problems, etc.).

A positive screen consists of a positive response to all four questions. Persons who sustained a traumatic brain injury and whose symptoms have since resolved are not identified using the VA clinical reminder. The requirement that the patient have experienced one or more related symptoms during the past week distinguishes the VA traumatic brain injury clinical reminder from other screening tools for traumatic brain injury, such as the BTBIS, which do not focus on current or persistent symptoms (Hill et al. 2009). Veterans who screen positive and who agree to further assessment or care are referred to a traumatic brain injury specialist or specialty clinic. In administering the VA traumatic brain injury clinical reminder, false positive errors can occur if current symptoms are due to other deployment-related conditions such as PTSD, depression, substance abuse, or chronic pain (Belanger et al. 2009). Nevertheless, other clinical reminders are in place for OEF/OIF/OND veterans seen at VA health care facilities including screening tools for PTSD, depression, and alcohol abuse.

Despite the need for brief screening tools for assessing mTBI from self-report, investigators have raised questions about the reliability and validity of information regarding brief alterations of consciousness obtained via self-report months or years after the fact (Belanger et al. 2009). In addition to traumatic brain injury, alterations of consciousness in combat may also result from acute stress, dissociation, sleep deprivation, or the general confusion of war (Hoge 2009). The lack of objective tests to identify mTBI poses challenges for health care providers who treat military service men and women and veterans who have had combat exposures. This has prompted increasing efforts to validate screening tools such as the VA traumatic brain injury clinical reminder, the BTBIS, and similar assessments used in non-veteran populations (Diamond et al. 2007; Schwab et al. 2007). A further issue is that dual diagnoses of mTBI and PTSD are frequent and the potential symptoms associated with each disorder partially overlap (Tanielian and Jaycox 2008). Distinguishing between the two conditions is likely to be important for identifying effective treatment approaches (Kupersmith et al. 2009). Although mTBI is predictive of a range of health problems, careful clinical evaluation is needed, since the primary problem may be PTSD or depression (Bryant 2008).

An increasing number of studies have examined the reliability and validity of the VA screening tool for TBI (Hill et al. 2009; Van Dyke et al. 2010; Donnelly et al. 2011). Hill et al. (2009) assessed the Department of Veterans Affairs screening tool for TBI by reviewing the medical records of 94 veterans seen in the VA Connecticut Healthcare System, from April 1, 2007 to March 30, 2008, who had screened positive for TBI and who had received clinical evaluation for the condition during the first year of the screening program. The majority of the veterans (85%) who screened positive met the American Congress of Rehabilitation Medicine definition of probable TBI. Hill et al. (2009) noted that, based solely upon results from the screening test, they had difficulty separating veterans with TBI alone from those who had both TBI and PTSD. Veterans with both PTSD and TBI reported more exposures and symptoms than veterans with a history of TBI and no PTSD (Hill 2009). Donnelly et al. (2011) examined the reliability, sensitivity, and specificity of the VA screening tool for TBI in 500 OEF/OIF veterans who underwent a structured diagnostic interview for TBI. The veterans were seen at five VA medical centers and one VA outpatient clinic in upstate New York. The screening tool had a high test-retest reliability (0.80), high sensitivity (0.94), and moderate specificity (0.59). However, the presence of PTSD symptoms (assessed using the PTSD checklist-military version) reduced the accuracy of the TBI screening tool (Donnelly et al. 2011). Van Dyke et al. (2010) examined the reliability of the VA TBI screening tool in a small sample of 33 OEF/OIF veterans. Preliminary findings from their study suggested poor overall test-retest reliability with respect to type of event, injuries sustained, and resulting sequelae (Van Dyke et al. 2010).

Clinical studies of civilians (for example, athletes) have found that the symptoms of cognitive effects of mTBI or concussion usually resolve within days to months (Levin et al. 1987; Iverson 2005; Schwab et al. 2007). However, as many as 10–20% of individuals with a mTBI have long-term *sequelae* for months or years after the injury (Alives et al. 1993; Hartlage et al. 2001; Vanderploeg et al. 2007). Precise estimates of the frequency of long-term *sequelae* following mTBI are lacking; studies have rarely considered associated injuries or comorbidities, and most studies have lacked comparison groups (Schwab et al. 2007).

In summary, current diagnostic procedures for TBI and PTSD in both military and civilian populations rely heavily on patient self-report, which is an important source of information in the diagnosis of most medical and psychiatric conditions. However, both TBI and PTSD can impact an individual's ability to recall or to communicate important aspects of the event. The inclusion of objective measures in diagnostic procedures for these conditions may increase accuracy and speed. Significant symptom overlap between TBI and PTSD presents another challenge for diagnosis. Identification of measures that could differentiate these conditions would facilitate diagnostic accuracy. Additional considerations, such as individual responses to exposures and symptoms may improve evaluation procedures as well. Accurate diagnosis is essential for appropriate treatment selection. Current treatments for TBI and PTSD are different, time-consuming, expensive, and can be emotionally draining for the patient. Finally, objective instruments, differential measures, and individual response information will increase our knowledge about these conditions, which may contribute to the discovery of more effective treatments.

STUDIES OF TRAUMATIC BRAIN INJURY AND PTSD

A sizeable number of studies have assessed both TBI and PTSD in military, veteran, and civilian populations. Studies of TBI among military populations differ from those of civilian populations in that all service members are employed at the time of injury and rates of substance abuse tend to be lower (Warden 2006). Some have found no differences between the *sequelae* of blast-related TBI and TBI resulting from non-combat causes such as motor vehicle accidents and falls (Belanger et al. 2009; Summers et al. 2009). However, the conditions under which war-related injuries occur are generally quite different from those of civilian injuries (Kupersmith et al. 2009). Previous authors have noted that PTSD may be more common among veterans with TBI than among civilians with TBI (Halbauer et al. 2009), although evidence to the contrary has also been provided (Tanielian and Jaycox 2008). Studies of TBI and PTSD in veteran populations are summarized in Table 8.1. Among those with military-related TBI, the frequency of probable PTSD varied widely across studies, which may reflect differences in study design, methods for assessing traumatic brain injury and PTSD, and selection factors. In three large studies that focused on OEF/OIF veterans, the frequencies of probable PTSD among those with mTBI ranged from 33% to 39% (Carlson et al. 2011).

Studies of TBI and PTSD in civilian populations are summarized in Table 8.2. These studies are summarized separate from those focusing on military populations because blast injuries—which are more common in combat situations—may involve different mechanical processes and different biological effects than those related to acceleration or deceleration injuries seen in motor vehicle accidents, falls, and sports. The results of these studies suggest that the incidence of PTSD among civilian TBI patients is about 13–27% (Bryant 1998; Turnbull et al. 2001; Creamer et al. 2005; Gil et al. 2005). However, estimates of the prevalence of PTSD in civilians who have suffered TBI vary dramatically (Kennedy et al. 2007).

The biological basis for a link between PTSD and traumatic brain injury may relate to shared exposures (for example, trauma from a blast injury or automobile accident). Biological models of PTSD may provide additional insight. For example, PTSD may involve an exaggerated response of the amygdala in the brain and impaired regulation of fear responses by the prefrontal cortex (Rauch et al. 2006; Bryant 2008). mTBI can involve damage to the prefrontal cortex due to shearing forces of the frontal regions of the brain against the cranium (Bryant 2008). It is possible that some individuals with mTBI may have an impaired ability to regulate fear reactions because of damage to neural networks that play a role in the regulation of fear and anxiety (Kennedy et al. 2007).

PTSD AND DEMENTIA

PTSD has been associated with numerous long-term health complications. Yaffe et al. (2010) found an increased risk of dementia in patients who had PTSD. Even after adjusting for demographics, neurological comorbidities, and general health comorbidities, those diagnosed with PTSD were 1.7 times more likely to experience dementia. The biological mechanisms that may account for a possible association between PTSD and dementia include pathophysiological mechanisms discussed in Chapters 6 and Chapter 7, such as alterations in hypothalamic-pituitary-adrenal axis hormones or proinflammatory cytokines. However, the specific neuropathological mechanisms that may account for a link between PTSD and dementia have not yet been identified. In chronic

Table 8.1.

Study	Sample	Study Design	Results	Limitations	Other Information
Koenigs et al. 2007	Vietnam veterans (n=193) with penetrating head injuries sustained during combat; veterans with combat exposure but no brain injury (n=52) who were evaluated for PTSD between April 2003 and November 2006 using the. Structured Clinical Interview (DSM-IV)	Clinical assessment of surviving members of a panel of veterans who had been previously studied in 1967–1970 and in 1981–1984.	PTSD was significantly reduced among those individuals with damage to one of two regions of the brain: the ventromedial prefrontal cortex ($p = 0.002$) and an anterior temporal area that included the amygdala, suggesting that these two areas are involved in the pathogenesis of PTSD. Although nearly half (48%) of the veterans in the non-brain-damaged group developed PTSD, only 18% of those in the ventrome-dial prefrontal cortex lesion group developed PTSD.	Combat exposure was greater for the brain-injured veterans than for the veterans without brain damage. Response bias was a potential limitation.	Data are from the Vietnam Head Injury Study and the study's registry.

(continued on next page)

Table 8.1. (*continued*)

Study	Sample	Study Design	Results	Limitations	Other Information
Vanderploeg et al. 2007	A sample of male Vietnam era veterans who served in the U.S. Army between January 1965 and December 1971. The veterans had undergone health evaluations in the mid-1980s. In the current analysis, the veterans were divided into those who had not been injured in a motor vehicle accident (MVA) since discharge from active duty nor had a mild traumatic brain injury (mTBI) (n=3,214), those who had been injured in a MVA but did not have a mTBI (n=539), and those who had a mTBI with altered consciousness (n=254).	Cross-sectional study conducted within an established cohort.	After controlling for demographic, prior or current medical conditions, and early-life psychiatric conditions (including anxiety disorder, mood disorder, conduct disorder, alcohol abuse, and other drug abuse prior to military service), no association was observed between generalized anxiety disorder or combat-related PTSD and group membership. Only 9 participants met criteria for accident-related PTSD, none of whom was in the mTBI group.	The study was limited to males. Information was lacking about additional head injuries prior to or during military service. No information was available about the date of the head injury or its severity. The cross-sectional nature of the study is a further limitation.	The data used for this study were from the Vietnam Experience Study. The participants were asked: "since your discharge from active duty, have you been injured in a motor vehicle accident?" They were also asked: "Since your discharge from active duty, have you injured your head?" And: "Did you lose consciousness as a result of the head injury."

(continued on next page)

Table 8.1. (continued)

Study	Sample	Study Design	Results	Limitations	Other Information
Vanderploeg et al. 2009	A sample of male Vietnam Era veterans who served in the U.S. Army between January 1965 and December 1971. The veterans had undergone health evaluations in the mid-1980s. In the current analysis, the veterans were divided into those who had not been injured in a MVA since discharge from activity duty nor had a mTBI (n=3,218), those who had been injured in a MVA but did not have a mTBI (n=558), and those who had a mTBI with altered consciousness (n=278).	Cross-sectional study conducted within an established cohort. This study was a reanalysis of data previously reported by Vanderploeg et al. (2007).	About 7.7% of the participants had current PTSD (within the last month). After controlling for demographic variables, combat intensity, medical conditions, and other current psychiatric conditions, mTBI was associated with a current diagnosis of PTSD. Overall, 11.5% of those who had sustained a mTBI had current PTSD as compared with 5.8% of MVA controls ($p < 0.01$). mTBI adversely affected long-term recovery from PTSD (odds ratio [OR] = 1.6, 95% confidence interval [CI] 1.1-2.4).	The study was limited to males. Information was lacking about additional head injuries prior to or during military service. No information was available about the date of the head injury or its severity. The cross-sectional nature of the study is a further limitation.	The data used for this study were from the Vietnam Experience Study.

(continued on next page)

Table 8.1. (continued)

Study	Sample	Study Design	Results	Limitations	Other Information
Schell and Marshall 2008	Men and women (n=1,965) in 24 targeted geographic areas of the U.S. who had been deployed to OEF/OIF.	Population-based telephone survey conducted between August 2007 and January 2008, with random digit dialing. PTSD was assessed using the Post-traumatic Symptom Checklist-Military Version. The BTBIS was used to assess probable TBI.	Based upon weighted percentages, 13.8% of the respondents had probable PTSD (95% CI 11.1%–16.5%) and 19.5% had probable TBI (95% CI 16.4%–22.7%). An estimated 1.1% (95% CI 0.6%–1.7%) had both probable PTSD and probable TBI.	The overall response rate was 44%. The BTBIS does not require current functional or cognitive impairment due to TBI. The analytic sample included 27 persons who volunteered to participate.	
Hoge et al. 2008	A sample of 2,525 U.S. Army infantry soldiers (95.5% male) who had returned from a year-long deployment to Iraq, 3–4 months prior to the survey.	Anonymous cross-sectional survey.	A total of 124 (4.9%) reported injuries with loss of consciousness and 260 (10.3%) reported injuries with altered mental status. About 43.9% of those reporting loss of consciousness met criteria for PTSD, as compared with 27.3% of those reporting altered mental status and 9.1% with no injury. After controlling for PTSD and depression, mTBI was not significantly associated with physical health outcomes or symptoms, except for headache.		The PTSD Checklist was used to assess PTSD. A three-question Defense and Veterans Brain Injury Center screening tool was used to assess TBI. The overall response rate was 59%.

(continued on next page)

Table 8.1. (continued)

Study	Sample	Study Design	Results	Limitations	Other Information
Ruff et al. 2008	Study of 126 veterans with mTBI associated with blast explosions who underwent neurological examination and neuropsychological testing at one VA medical center.	Clinical study.	The frequency of PTSD was 90% among veterans with neurocognitive deficits and 24% among those without neurocognitive deficits ($p < .001$, OR = 28.6, 95% CI 10.6–77.6).	Small sample size. The generalizability of the results is uncertain.	The main focus of this study was on headaches. The PTSD checklist (PCL-17) was used to assess PTSD.
Hill et al. 2009	Combat Veterans (n=94) in the VA Connecticut Healthcare System who both screened positive for TBI and received clinical evaluation for TBI between April 1, 2007 and March 30, 2008.	Retrospective evaluation study	All but one case were classified as mTBI. About 35% of those with TBI had PTSD. Veterans with both PTSD and TBI were more likely to report falling as a mechanism of injury and indicated they had suffered a head injury during deployment ($p < 0.10$).	Small sample size.	
Schneiderman et al. 2009	Male and female OEF/OIF veterans (n=2,235) who had left combat theatres by September 2004 and lived in Maryland, northern Virginia, Washington, DC, and eastern West Virginia.	Cross-sectional postal survey.	About 12% of the 2,235 respondents reported a history consistent with mTBI and 11% screened positive for PTSD.	The response rate was 35%. The respondents may not have been fully representative of OEF/OIF veterans.	PTSD was assessed using the PTSD Checklist-Civilian Version. The three-item BTBIS was also used.

(continued on next page)

Table 8.1. (*continued*)

Study	Sample	Study Design	Results	Limitations	Other Information
Pietrzak et al. (2009)	A sample of 277 Connecticut veterans of OEF/OIF between January 1, 2003 and March 1, 2007. The participants were predominantly white and male.	Cross-sectional survey conducted in October 2007.	About 18.8% (52 of 277) of the sample screened positive for mTBI. Those with mTBI were more likely to meet screening criteria for PTSD. PTSD mediated the relationship between mTBI and other outcomes (unmet medical and psychological needs and perceived barriers to care).	The response rate was 28.5%. Respondents were older than non-respondents in the sampling frame (33.4 versus. 31.3 years, $p = 0.004$). The sample size was small overall.	The PTSD checklist-Military version was used to assess PTSD. The VA screening questionnaire for TBI was used.
Nelson et al. 2009	OEF/OIF veterans, 35 with TBI and 19 with both TBI and PTSD.	Case-control analysis of cognitive tests.	Measures of processing speed accounted for a significant portion of executive performance in both TBI, and TBI/PTSD groups. Cognitive flexibility was similar between the two groups. However, response inhibition and color-naming speed were significantly reduced in the TBI/PTSD group.	Small sample size, high variation in time since injury, and uncertain generalizability of results.	

(continued on next page)

Table 8.1. (*continued*)

Study	Sample	Study Design	Results	Limitations	Other Information
Campbell et al. 2009	A sample of 70 OEF/OIF combat veterans with PTSD, TBI, or both.	Analysis of subset of data from prior research.	The TBI/PTSD group had significantly longer time since injury (28.4 months) than the TBI alone group (9.7 months). The PTSD and PTSD/TBI groups both performed worse on the Stroop Color/Word test than the TBI group. The TBI/PTSD group performed worse than the PTSD group on the Stroop Color score. TBI alone did not account for worse neuropsychological outcomes than PTSD alone on any of the executive performance or processing speed measures.	Mechanism of blast and presence of depression were not analyzed. No healthy controls were included.	

(continued on next page)

Table 8.1. (*continued*)

Study	Sample	Study Design	Results	Limitations	Other Information
Brenner et al. (2010)	Injured soldiers (n = 1,247) from one Fort Carson Brigade Combat Team in Colorado.	Cross-sectional analysis of data from Post Deployment Health Assessment.	A total of 878 (71%) of the soldiers had mTBI, 405 (33%) screened positive for PTSD, and 323 (26%) had mTBI and screened positive for PTSD. After controlling for age, gender, education, rank, and military occupational specialty, PTSD and mTBI together were more strongly associated with having post-concussive symptoms (adjusted prevalence ratio [PR] = 6.3, 95% CI 4.1–9.4) than either mTBI alone (PR = 4.0, 95% CI 2.7–6.1) or PTSD alone (PR = 2.7, 95% CI 1.6–4.7).	The generalizability of the results is uncertain.	TBI was assessed using the Warrior Administered Retrospective Casualty Assessment Tool (WARCAT) which is based on the BTBIS. After completing the WARCAT, soldiers were interviewed by clinicians.

(continued on next page)

Table 8.1. (*continued*)

Study	Sample	Study Design	Results	Limitations	Other Information
Kennedy et al. 2010	Samples of 586 OEF/OIF service members with blast-related mTBI and 138 OEF/OIF service members with non-blast mTBI.	Retrospective review of research records.	Reexperiencing symptoms such as flashbacks and nightmares were higher for the blast mTBI group than for the non-blast mTBI group. Using a cut-off score of 50 on the PCL-C, 37.3% of the total sample showed elevated scores. The percentages of the blast and non-blast groups with a PCL-C score of 50 or greater did not significantly differ (38.2% vs. 33.3%, respectively, $p = 0.29$).	The sample size was small for some analyses. The blast and non-blast groups differed by age, gender, and branch of service.	PTSD was assessed using the PTSD Checklist-Civilian Version
MacGregor et al. 2010	A sample of 781 men injured during military combat in Iraq between September 2004 and February 2005.	Review of U.S. Navy-Marine Corps Combat Trauma Registry Expeditionary Medical Encounter Database (CTR-EMED)	About 15.8% met criteria for TBI (13.4% mild, 2.4% moderate to severe), 35.0% had other head injury, and 49.2% had non-head injury. In the overall cohort, the rate of PTSD was 16.5%. About 12.4% (13 of 105) of the men with mTBI had PTSD.	The study assessed only provider-diagnosed TBI documented in clinical records from the point of injury. This study was limited to men.	A diagnosis of PTSD was indicated by an ICD-9 code 309.81. PTSD diagnosis must have been made at least 1 month post-injury. TBI was defined using CTR-EMED clinical records after review by CTR-EMED clinical research staff.

(continued on next page)

Table 8.1. *(continued)*

Study	Sample	Study Design	Results	Limitations	Other Information
Carlson et al. 2010	Review of records of 13,201 U.S. military veterans who were screened for traumatic brain injury in VA health care facilities in the Upper Midwest Integrated Service Network between April 1, 2007 and October 20, 2008.	Analysis of VA administrative records	Veterans with positive screens for TBI (n = 2,279) were 3 times more likely to have a PTSD diagnosis (relative risk = 3.3, 95% CI 3.1 – 3.5). Among veterans with a positive TBI screen, those with clinically confirmed TBI (n = 836) were more likely to have PTSD than those without confirmed TBI status (63.9% vs. 60.8%, respectively).	Limitations include use of VA administrative data rather than structured clinical interviews to identify those with TBI. The use of ICD-9 codes to identify PTSD may also have introduced some misclassification.	
Lippa et al. 2010	A sample of 339 OEF/OIF veterans with mTBI histories who were evaluated as outpatients at two VA medical centers as part of comprehensive TBI evaluation.	Information was obtained from self-report forms completed at the time of the evaluation. Semi-structured interviews were also conducted by a medical provider.	On average, veterans with any blast-related mTBI history were younger and reported higher posttraumatic stress symptoms than those with nonblast-related mTBI histories. Post-traumatic stress symptoms accounted for a substantial portion (46.6%) of variance in reported post-concussive symptoms.	Veterans with no history of mTBI were not included in the study. Data were based upon self-report.	On average, 3 years had elapsed since the veterans' most recent injuries.

(continued on next page)

Table 8.1. (*continued*)

Study	Sample	Study Design	Results	Limitations	Other Information
Polusny et al. 2011	The participants were 953 U.S. National Guard soldiers (92.5% male) surveyed in Iraq 1 month before returning home (time 1) and 1 year later (time 2).	In this longitudinal cohort study, the time 1 sample was assessed during redeployment transition briefings held at military installations in the Iraq combat theater. The time 2 sample was assessed using mailed surveys sent to the homes of U.S. National Guard service members.	The rate of self-reported mTBI during deployment was 9.2% at time 1 and 22.0% at time 2. At time 1, 7.6% of the panel met screening criteria for PTSD. A higher percentage (18.2%) met criteria for PTSD at time 2. Time 1 PTSD symptoms more strongly predicted post-deployment symptoms and outcomes than did history of concussion or mTBI. PTSD was strongly associated with post-concussive symptoms 1 year after soldiers returned from Iraq.	Differences in rates of reported mTBI between time 1 and time 2 could be the result of recall bias or different contexts for assessment. Non-combat TBI was not asked about. Response bias is also a possibility.	This is the first study to assess soldiers' report of concussion and mTBI while in theater and to longitudinally examine the impact of concussion and mTBI 1 year following return from combat deployment.

Table 8.2.

Study	Sample	Study Design	Results	Limitations	Other Information
Middelboe et al. 1992	51 patients (33 males, 18 females) admitted to a hospital in Denmark after minor head injury, resulting from traffic accidents (49%), falls (33%), assault (12%), and other causes (6%).	Prospective follow-up study involving semi-structured interviews, self-administered questionnaires, and symptom checklists. The patients were assessed at 1 week and 3 months.	Nearly half of the patients (46%) had considerable discomfort at 1 week. The incidence of PTSD was low (1 of 51 or 2%).	Small sample size. Lack of a comparison group. Possible selection bias and uncertain generalizability of results.	The Impact of Event Scale was used to assess intrusion and avoidance symptoms. PTSD was defined according to DSM-III-R criteria. The study completion rate was 75%.
Alexander 1992	Outpatients (n = 36) who were referred for persistent neurologic symptoms >6 months after mild closed head injury.	Clinical interview, mental status examination, and neurologic examination.	Only 1 of 36 patients met criteria for PTSD.	Small sample size. Lack of comparison group. Possible selection bias and uncertain generalizability of results.	Patients who had received inpatient rehabilitation treatment were excluded along with those who had not undergone neuroimaging.
Ohry et al. 1996	Outpatients (n = 24) with head injuries who were treated in a rehabilitation program in Long Island, New York.	Standardized questionnaires were used to collect information from the participants, 6 to 8 months following their injuries.	33% (8 of 24) met criteria for PTSD.	Small sample size. Lack of comparison group. Inclusion of patients with cerebral vascular accident (n = 11) was also a limitation. Possible selection bias and uncertain generalizability of results.	The PTSD Inventory based on DSM-III-R criteria was used to assess PTSD.

(continued on next page)

Table 8.2. (continued)

Study	Sample	Study Design	Results	Limitations	Other Information
Grigsby and Kaye 1993	The sample included 70 persons who had sustained head injuries and were referred for neuropsychological assessment.	Clinical interviews and neuropsychological testing.	About 50% (35 of 70) had experienced feelings of unreality following their injuries. Only 11% (2 of 18) of those with a period of unconsciousness ≥30 minutes had similar complaints. About 51% of those who complained of feelings of unreality also met DSM-III-R criteria for PTSD.	Small sample size. Lack of a comparison group. Possible selection bias and uncertain generalizability of results.	The Structured Clinical Interview for DSM-III-R Dissociative Disorders was used.
Hickling et al. 1998	107 MVA survivors (some with mTBI) who were referred for neuropsychological testing.	12 month follow-up study. Initial assessments were completed 1–4 months post-injury.	About 36% (38 of 107) had PTSD. The frequency of PTSD did not significantly differ according to whether the participants had whiplash or struck their head, or lost consciousness.	Small sample size. Lack of a comparison group. Possible selection bias and uncertain generalizability of results.	PTSD was assessed using the Clinician-Administered PTSD Scale.

(continued on next page)

Table 8.2. (*continued*)

Study	Sample	Study Design	Results	Limitations	Other Information
Hibbard et al. 1998	A sample of 100 community-dwelling adults with TBI, living in New York State, who were between 18 and 65 years of age; 53% male, 47% female. All participants had a TBI of any severity at least 1 year prior to the interview.	Retrospective survey involving structured interviews. PTSD and other Axis I diagnoses were determined for 3 time points (pre-TBI, post-TBI, and current diagnosis).	About 6% (6 of 100) had PTSD prior to their injuries; 19% had PTSD following their injuries. Little resolution of PTSD was observed over time.	Study limitations include the retrospective assessment of diagnoses. Individuals with more severe TBI may have underreported some symptoms.	The Structured Clinical Interview for DSM-IV Diagnoses was used. The majority of brain injuries (62%) were caused by MVAs.
Bryant and Harvey 1998	79 adults with mTBI who were admitted to a trauma hospital in Sydney, Australia following a MVA.	Follow-up study involving initial assessments 2 to 28 days post-injury and 6 month follow-up interviews.	6 Months post-injury 24% (15 of 63) met criteria for PTSD.	The follow-up rate at 6 months was 80% (63 of 79). Small sample size. Lack of a comparison group. Possible selection bias and uncertain generalizability of results.	At follow-up, PTSD was assessed using the PTSD module of the Composite International Diagnostic Interview.

(continued on next page)

Table 8.2. (continued)

Study	Sample	Study Design	Results	Limitations	Other Information
Bryant and Harvey 1999	Patients with mTBI (n = 46) and no traumatic brain injury (n = 59) who were admitted to a trauma hospital in Sydney, Australia following a MVA.	Interviews were conducted 6 months post-injury.	Post-concussive symptoms were more evident in mTBI patients with PTSD than those without PTSD, and in mTBI patients than non-traumatic brain injury patients. At 6-months post trauma, 20% (9 of 46) of the patients with mTBI had PTSD as compared to 25% (15 of 59) of the non-traumatic brain injury patients.	Small sample size. Possible selection bias and uncertain generalizability of results.	The PTSD module of the Composite International Diagnostic Interview was used along with a Post-concussive Symptom Checklist.
Bryant et al. 2000a, 2000b	96 adults (77 male, 19 female) with severe traumatic brain injury who were admitted to rehabilitation hospital in Sydney, Australia.	Structured clinical interviews were conducted 5–7 months post-injury.	PTSD was diagnosed in 27% (26 of 96) of the patients.	Small sample size. Lack of a comparison group. Possible selection bias and uncertain generalizability of results.	Clinical assessment of PTSD was based on DSM-III-R criteria.

(continued on next page)

Table 8.2. (*continued*)

Study	Sample	Study Design	Results	Limitations	Other Information
Turnbull et al. 2001	53 persons with TBI identified using accident and emergency unit records in Scotland.	Cross-sectional study involving structured clinical interviews.	The frequency of PTSD was between 17% (11 of 41) and 27% (7 of 41). Having amnesia for the traumatic incident was associated with a decreased severity of PTSD symptoms.	Small sample size. Lack of a comparison group. The response rate was only 15%. Possible selection bias and uncertain generalizability of results.	Persons with chronic alcohol abuse were excluded. The revised Impact of Events Scale was used to assess PTSD. The Clinician-administered PTSD scale for DSM-IV was also used.
Levin et al. 2001	69 patients (49 male, 20 female) with mild (n = 60) or moderate (n = 9) TBI, along with 52 extracranial trauma patient controls, seen at a trauma center in Houston.	Follow-up study with an assessment 3 months post-injuries.	About 13% (8 of 60) patients with mTBI and none of the 9 patients with ModTBI had PTSD 3 months post injuries. In the extracranial trauma group, 12% (6 of 52) met diagnostic criteria for PTSD.	Small sample size. Possible selection bias and uncertain generalizability of results.	Patients with a penetrating injury to the brain were excluded, along with those with a history of schizophrenia, hospitalization for previous TBI, history of treatment for recent substance abuse, or a blood alcohol level ≥ 200 mg/dL. PTSD was diagnosed using the Structured Clinical Interview for DSM-IV.

(continued on next page)

Table 8.2. *(continued)*

Study	Sample	Study Design	Results	Limitations	Other Information
Hoofien et al. 2001	76 persons (63 male, 13 female) who had suffered severe TBI were evaluated an average of 14.1 years post injuries.	Follow-up study of persons referred to a community-based, neuropsychological rehabilitation center in Jerusalem.	About 14% of the sample had chronic PTSD.	Possible attrition bias. Lack of a comparison group.	About 50% of the patients eligible for the study were not located. PTSD was assessed using the PTSD Inventory following DSM-III criteria.
Williams et al. 2002a, 2002b	Community sample of 66 survivors (50 male and 16 female) of severe TBI. A total of 51 had been in road accidents, 12 had suffered falls, 2 had been physically assaulted, and 1 had been injured in a bomb explosion.	Clinical evaluation 1 to 26 years (mean = 5.9 years, SD 4.9 years) post injuries.	About 18% had moderate to severe PTSD symptoms.	Small sample size. Lack of a comparison group.	The Impact of Events inventory was used to assess PTSD symptoms.

(continued on next page)

Table 8.2. (*continued*)

Study	Sample	Study Design	Results	Limitations	Other Information
Glaesser et al. 2004	Sample of 46 inpatients (32 male, 14 female) who had suffered a traumatic brain or cervical spine injury who were treated at a neurological rehabilitation clinic in Germany. About 27% of the patients had been unconscious for ≥12 hours.	Cross-sectional study involving clinical interviews.	About 27% (4 of 15) of the patients who had not been unconscious following their injury, or had only been unconscious for a few minutes to 1 hour, met criteria for PTSD. Only 3% (1 of 31) of those who had been unconscious for ≥12 hours had PTSD.	Small sample size. Possible selection bias and uncertain generalizability of results.	PTSD was assessed using the Structured Clinical Interview for DSM-IV (German version).
Ashman et al. 2004	188 persons who had sustained TBI < 4 years of enrollment into the study (29% mild, 62% moderate to severe, and 9% with loss of consciousness of unknown duration.)	Cross-sectional and longitudinal study designs. The participants underwent 2 to 3 assessments. Each assessment was about 1 year apart. Of the 188 participants, 83 completed the third assessment.	Rates of PTSD were 30% at the time of the first assessment and declined to 18% and 21% by the time of the second and third assessments.	Possible attrition bias.	PTSD was assessed using the Structured Clinical Interview for DSM-IV.

(continued on next page)

Table 8.2. (*continued*)

Study	Sample	Study Design	Results	Limitations	Other Information
Jones et al. 2005	131 persons (40% male, 60% female) who did (n=66) and did not (n=65) sustain mild or moderate TBI following a MVA or other road accident. The patients were seen in the emergency department of a hospital in Oxford, Great Britain.	Follow-up study with initial assessment followed by assessments at 6 weeks and 3 months post-trauma.	At the initial assessment, those with TBI reported more fear and helplessness at the time of the trauma, and more recurrent intrusive thoughts and images, and dissociation. At 3 months post trauma, there was no difference in the pattern of PTSD symptomatology between the TBI and non-TBI groups. About 17% (10 of 58) of the persons with mTBI had PTSD 3 months post trauma compared to 69% (11 of 16) of the non-TBI group.	Small sample size. Possible selection bias and uncertain generalizability of results.	PTSD was assessed using the interview version of the PTSD Symptom Scale.
Sumpter and McMillan 2005	34 persons (30 male and 4 female) with severe traumatic brain injury recruited from community services in Glascow, UK.	Self-administered questionnaire followed by a structured clinical interview.	Based upon questionnaires, 44% to 59% of the participants met screening criteria for PTSD. However, only 3% (1 of 34) had PTSD based upon structured clinical interviews.	Small sample size. Possible selection bias and uncertain generalizability of results.	PTSD was assessed using self-administered screening questionnaires (Post-traumatic Diagnostic Scale and Impact of Events Scale) and using the Clinician-Administered PTSD Scale.

(continued on next page)

Table 8.2. (continued)

Study	Sample	Study Design	Results	Limitations	Other Information
Gil et al. 2005	A total of 123 persons (58% male, 42% female) with mTBI who were recruited from 2 surgical wards at a medical center in Israel.	Follow-up study with assessments immediately after the traumatic event and follow-up at 1 week, 3 months, and 6 months. Self-administered questionnaires were combined with clinical interviews.	Overall, 14% (17 of 120) of the participants met criteria for PTSD at 6 months. Those with memory of the traumatic event were more likely to develop PTSD than those without memory of the event.	Of 198 eligible person, 44 (23%) refused to participate and 34 (17%) dropped out during the follow-up period. Possible selection bias and uncertain generalizability of results.	PTSD was assessed using the Clinician-Administered PTSD Scale and the Posttraumatic Stress Scale.
Creamer et al. 2005	307 consecutive patients (77% male, 23% female) admitted to a trauma center in Melbourne, Australia for at least 24 hours.	Follow-up study involving structured clinical interviews.	About 62% (n = 189) of the participants met criteria for mTBI. Over 10% (n = 32) of participants had PTSD by 12 months post-injury. PTSD was more frequent among those with mTBI but the difference was not statistically significant. Non-significant differences were observed in the incidence of PTSD between those with full recall of the event (9%), partial recall (14%), and no recall of the event (7%).	A total of 307 individuals completed the 12-month assessment (85% retention rate). Limited sample size for some comparisons. Uncertain generalizability of results.	PTSD was assessed at 12 months post-injury using the Clinician-Administered PTSD Scale.

(continued on next page)

Table 8.2. (continued)

Study	Sample	Study Design	Results	Limitations	Other Information
Greenspan et al. 2006	Convenience sample of 198 persons (66% male) with TBI (19% mild, 21% moderate, and 60% severe) who were discharged from participating rehabilitation hospitals in Georgia and North Carolina. The main causes of injury included motor vehicle crash (70%), fall (16%), and pedestrian injury (6%).	Follow-up study. Telephone interviews were completed at 6 months and 12 months post-injury.	PTSD symptoms increased from 11% at 6 months to 16% at 12 months post-injury. Women reported greater PTSD symptomatology than men. TBI severity and memory of the event were not associated with PTSD symptoms.	A total of 78 participants were excluded from the analysis because they were missing either the 6 or 12 month Impact of Event Scale score. Study limitations include the lack of clinical assessment of PTSD, possible selection bias, and uncertain generalizability of results.	PTSD symptoms were assessed using the Impact of Event Scale.
Whelan-Goodinson et al. 2009	100 persons who suffered a TBI 6 months to 5.5 years previously who were referred to a rehabilitation center in Melbourne, Australia. Most of the patients had suffered moderate to severe TBI.	Cross-sectional survey.	About 10% (10 of 100) developed PTSD post-injury; 4% (4 of 100) had PTSD at the time of their injury.	Limited sample size for some comparisons. Possible selection bias and uncertain generalizability of results. Retrospective ascertainment of PTSD.	The Structured Clinical Interview for DSM-IV Disorders was used to assess PTSD. A "significant other" was also interviewed in 87% of the cases.

(continued on next page)

Table 8.2. (*continued*)

Study	Sample	Study Design	Results	Limitations	Other Information
Bryant et al. 2010	Patients (n = 1,084) recently admitted to 4 trauma hospitals in Australia. Persons with moderate or severe brain injury were excluded. About 40% (437 of 1,084) had mTBI.	Prospective cohort study involving initial assessments during hospital admission and telephone follow-up interviews at 3 months (n=932, 86%) and 12 months (n=817, 75%) post-injury.	Among patients with mTBI who participated in the 3 month follow-up interview, about 13% (48 of 377) had PTSD. The rate of new diagnoses of PTSD was about 7% (28 of 377) at 12 months.	Of 1,477 trauma patients who met inclusion criteria, 1,084 (73%) agreed to participate. Possible selection bias.	Patients who declined to participate in the study did not differ from participants in gender, length of hospital admission, injury severity score, or age. The Mini International Neuropsychiatric Interview was used to assess PTSD in hospital. The Clinician-Administered PTSD Scale for DSM-IV was used to assess PTSD at the 3 and 12 month follow-up interviews.

traumatic encephalopathy, a potential late complication of head injuries sustained during contact sports such as boxing and football (Costanza et al. 2011), the important exposure is multiple blows to the head rather than a traumatic psychological event. Nevertheless, because some persons with a lifetime history of PTSD may have experienced repeated physical assault, battering, or combat-related TBI, longitudinal studies of PTSD and dementia should strive to differentiate between dementia, chronic traumatic encephalopathy, and Alzheimer's disease.

SUMMARY AND CONCLUSIONS

This review of the literature on TBI and PTSD in military, veteran, and civilian populations highlights the importance of brain injuries from both public health and clinical perspectives. There has been extended recent discussion over how best to identify and treat mTBI among returning combat veterans and other populations, especially in situations where brain injury may overlap with PTSD (Belanger et al. 2009; Bryant 2008; Hill et al. 2009; Hoge et al. 2009; Carlson et al. 2011). There are likely many opportunities to intervene to assist persons with traumatic brain injury through the development of improved screening and diagnostic tools, multidisciplinary health care teams and integrated systems of care, amelioration of current or persisting symptoms and comorbid conditions, family support, public and professional education, and provision of job training, educational, and/or rehabilitative services. For an individual patient, the need for each of these components is likely to change or evolve over time.

Additional basic research and clinical translational research are needed. Based upon a systematic review of the literature, Carlson et al. (2011) recommended that researchers strive to reach a consensus about how best to define and measure both TBI and PTSD so that these practices can be consistently applied across studies. They also recommended studies of the negative and positive predictive values of PTSD assessment methods among veterans with a history of mTBI (Carlson et al. 2011). Ongoing studies in veteran populations are examining whether TBI induces subtle lesions in the emotional-regulatory pathway that may manifest themselves as PTSD (Kupersmith et al. 2009). Prior studies have suggested that PTSD may be associated with dysfunction of the prefrontal cortex, hippocampus, and amygdala (Bremner et al. 2008; Koenigs et al. 2008). Additional research is also needed to identify neuroimaging markers that distinguish TBI from PTSD (Kupersmith et al. 2009). Furthermore, follow-up studies are also needed to better understand the post-acute and long-term outcomes of psychological and neurological outcomes of combat-related TBI.

REFERENCES

Alexander MP. 1992. Neuropsychiatric correlates of persistent postconcussive syndrome. *J Head Trauma Rehabil.* 7:60–69.

Alves W, Macciocchi SN, Barth JT. 1993. Postconcussive symptoms after uncomplicated mild head injury. *J Head Trauma Rehabil.* 8:48–59.

Ashman TA, Spielman LA, Hibbard MR, et al. 2004. Psychiatric challenges in the first 6 years after traumatic brain injury: cross-sequential analyses of Axis I disorders. *Arch Phys Med Rehabil.* 85:36–42.

Belanger HG, Oomoto JM, Vanderploeg RD. 2009. The Veterans Health Administration system of care for mild traumatic brain injury: costs, benefits, and controversies. *J Health Trauma Rehabil.* 24:4–13.

Bhattacharjee Y. 2008. Neuroscience. Shell shock revisited: solving the puzzle of blast trauma. *Science.* 319:406–408.

Bowe M. 2007. The Evolution of trauma resucitation in a combat support hospital. *Journal of Emergency Nursing.* 33(1):83–86.

Bremner JD, Elzinga B, Schmahl C, et al. 2008. Structural and functional plasticity of the human brain in posttraumatic stress disorder. *Prog Brain Res.* 167:171–186.

Brenner LA, Ivins BJ, Schwab K, et al. 2010. Posttraumatic stress disorder, and postconcussive symptom reporting among troops returning from Iraq. *J Head Trauma Rehabil.* 25:307–312.

Bryant RA, Harvey AG. 1999. Postconcussive symptoms and posttraumatic stress disorder after mild traumatic brain injury. *J Nervous Mental Dis.* 187:302–305.

Bryant RA. 2008. Disentangling mild traumatic brain injury and stress reactions. *N Engl J Med.* 358:525–527.

Bryant RA, Harvey AG. 1998. Relationship between acute stress disorder and posttraumatic stress disorder following mild traumatic brain injury. *Am J Psychiatry*. 1155:625–629.

Bryant RA, Harvey AG. 1999. The influence of traumatic brain injury on acute stress disorder and post-traumatic stress disorder following motor vehicle accidents. *Brain Injury*. 13:15–22.

Bryant RA, Marosszeky JE, Crooks J, Gurka JA. 2000a. Posttraumatic stress disorder after severe traumatic brain injury. *Am J Psychiatry*. 157:629–631.

Bryant RA, Marosszeky JE, Crooks J, et al. 2000b. Coping style and post-traumatic stress disorder following severe traumatic brain injury. *Brain Inj*. 14:175–180.

Bryant RA, Harvey AG. 1999. Postconcussive symptoms and posttraumatic stress disorder after mild traumatic brain injury. *J Nervous Mental Dis*. 187:302–305.

Bryant RA, O'Donnell ML, Creamer M, et al. 2010. The psychiatric sequelae of traumatic injury. *Am J Psychiatry*. 167:312–320.

Butler D, Buono J, Erdtmann F, Reid P, editors. 2008. *Systems Engineering to Improve Traumatic Brain Injury Care in the Military Health System*. Washington, DC: National Academies Press.

Carlson KF, Kehle SM, Meis LA, et al. 2011. Prevalence, assessment, and treatment of mild traumatic brain injury and posttraumatic stress disorder: a systematic review of the evidence. *J Head Trauma Rehabil*. 26:103–115.

Carlson KF, Nelson D, Orazem RJ, et al. 2010. Psychiatric diagnoses among Iraq and Afghanistan War veterans screened for deployment-related traumatic brain injury. *J Trauma Stress*. 23:17–24.

Cernak I, Noble-Haeusslein LJ. 2010. Traumatic brain injury: an overview of pathobiology with emphasis on military populations. *J Cereb Blood Flow Metab*. 30(2):255–266.

Chapman JC, Andersen AM, Roselli LA, et al. 2010. Screening for mild traumatic brain injury in the presence of psychiatric comorbidities. *Arch Phys Med Rehabil*. 91(7):1082–1086.

Collins M, Lovell M, Iverson G, et al. 2002. Cumulative effects of concussion in high school athletes. *Neurosurgery*. 51:1175–1181.

Costanza A, Weber K, Gandy S, et al. 2011. Contact sport-related traumatic encephalopathy in the elderly: clinical expression and structural substrates. *Neuropathol Appl Neurobiol.* 37:570–584.

Courtney AC, Courtney MW. 2009. A thoracic mechanism of mild traumatic brain injury due to blast pressure waves. *Med Hypotheses.* 72(1):76–83.

Creamer M, O'Donnell ML, Pattison P. 2005. Amnesia, traumatic brain injury, and posttraumatic stress disorder: a methodological inquiry. *Behav Res Ther.* 43:1383–1389.

DeKosky ST, Ikonomovic MD, Gandy S. 2010. Traumatic brain injury—football, warfare, and long-term effects. *N Engl J Med.* 363:1293–1296.

DePalma RG, Burris DG, Champion HR, et al. 2005. Blast injuries. *N Engl J Med.* 352:1335–1342.

Department of Veterans Affairs Traumatic Brain Injury: Independent Study Course 2010: Department of Veterans Affairs Employee Education System.

Diamond PM, Harzke AJ, Magaletta PR, et al. 2007. Screening for traumatic brain injury in an offender sample: a first look at the reliability and validity of the Traumatic Brain Injury Questionnaire. *J Head Trauma Rehabil.* 22:330–338.

Donnelly KT, Donnelly JP, Dunnam M, et al. 2011. Reliability, sensititivity, and specificity of the VA Traumatic Brain Injury Screening Tool. *J Head Trauma Rehabil.* 26:439–453.

Faul M, Xu L, Wald MM, Coronado VG. 2010. Traumatic brain injury in the United States: emergency department visits, hospitalizations, and deaths. Atlanta, GA: Centers for Disease Control and Prevention. Available at: http://www.cdc.gov/TraumaticBrainInjury/index.html Accessed January 21, 2012

Faux S, Sheedy J, Delaney R, et al. 2011. Emergency department prediction of post-concussive syndrome following mild traumatic brain injury–an international cross-validation study. *Brain Inj.* 25(1):14–22.

Galarneau MR, Woodruff SI, Dye JL, et al. 2008. Traumatic brain injury during Operation Iraqi Freedom: findings from the United States Navy-Marine Corps Combat Trauma Registry. *J Neurosurg.* 108:950–957.

Gil S, Caspi Y, Ben-Ari IZ, et al. 2005. Does memory of a traumatic event increase the risk for posttraumatic stress disorder in patients with traumatic brain injury? A prospective study. *Am J Psychiatry.* 162:963–969.

Glaesser J, Neuner F, Lutgehetmann R, et al. 2004. Posttraumatic stress disorder in patients with traumatic brain injury. *BMC Psychiatry.* 4:5.

Greenspan AI, Stringer AY, Phillips VL, et al. 2006. Symptoms of post-traumatic stress: intrusion and avoidance 6 and 12 months after TBI. *Brain Inj.* 20:733–742.

Grigsby J, Kaye K. 1993. Incidence and correlates of depersonalization following head trauma. *Brain Injury.* 7:507–513.

Guskiewicz K, McCrea M, Marshall S, et al. 2003. Cumulative effects associated with recurrent concussion in collegiate football players. *JAMA.* 290(19):2549–2555.

Halbauer JD, Ashford JW, Zeitzer JM, et al. 2009. Neuropsychiatric diagnosis and management of chronic sequelae of war-related mild to moderate traumatic brain injury. *J Rehab Res Dev.* 46:757–796.

Han SD, Suzuki H, Drake AI, et al. 2009. Clinical, cognitive, and genetic predictors of change in job status following traumatic brain injury in a military population. *J Head Trauma Rehabil.* 24:57–64.

Hartlage LC, Durant-Wilson D, Patch PC. 2001. Persistent neurobehavioral problems following mild traumatic brain injury. *Arch Clin Neuropsychol.* 16:561–570.

Hellawell DJ, Taylor R, Pentland, B. 1999. Cognitive and psychosocial outcome following moderate or severe traumatic brain injury. *Brain Injury.* 13(7): 489–504.

Hibbard MR, Uysal S, Kepler K, et al. 1998. Axis I psychopathology in individuals with traumatic brain injury. *J Head Trauma Rehabil.* 13:24–39.

Hicks RR, Fertig SJ, Desrocher RE, et al. 2010. Neurological effects of blast injury. *J Trauma.* 68(5):1257–1263.

Hickling EJ, Gillen R, Blanchard EB, et al. 1998. Traumatic brain injury and posttraumatic stress disorder: a preliminary investigation of neuropsychological test results in PTSD secondary to motor vehicle accidents. *Brain Inj.* 12:265–274.

Hill JJ III, Mobo BHP Jr, Cullen MR. 2009. Separating deployment-related traumatic brain injury and posttraumatic stress disorder in veterans. Preliminary findings from the Veterans Affairs Traumatic Brain Injury Screening Program. *Am J Phys Med Rehabil.* 88:605–614.

Hoge CW, Auchterloine JL, Milliken CS. 2006. Mental health problems, use of mental health services, and attrition from military service after returning from deployment to Iraq or Afghanistan. *JAMA.* 295:1023–1032.

Hoge CW, Goldberg HM, Castro CA. 2009. Care of war veterans with mild traumatic brain injury—flawed perspectives (commentary). *N Engl J Med.* 360:1588–1591.

Hoge CW, McGurk D, Thomas JL, et al. 2008. Mild traumatic brain injury in U.S. Soldiers returning from Iraq. *N Engl J Med.* 358(5):453–463.

Hoofien D, Gilboa A, Vakil E, Donovick PJ. 2001. Traumatic brain injury (TBI) 10–20 years later: a comprehensive outcome study of psychiatric symptomatology, cognitive abilities and psychosocial functioning. *Brain Inj.* 15:189–209.

Iverson GL. 2005. Outcome from mild traumatic brain injury. *Curr Opin Psychiatry.* 18:301–317.

Jones C, Harvey AG, Brewin CR. 2005. Traumatic brain injury, dissociation, and posttraumatic stress disorder in road traffic accident survivors. *J Trauma Stress.* 18:181–191.

Kennedy JE, Jaffee MS, Leskin GA, et al. 2007. Posttraumatic stress disorder and posttraumatic stress disorder-like symptoms and mild traumatic brain injury. *J Rehabil Res Dev.* 44:895–920.

Kennedy JE, Leal FO, Lewis JD, et al. 2010. Posttraumatic stress symptoms in OIF/OEF service members with blast-related and non-blast-related mild TBI. *Neuro Rehabilitation.* 26:223–231.

Koenigs M, Huey ED, Raymont V, et al. 2008. Focal brain damage protects against post-traumatic stress disorder in combat veterans. *Nat Neurosci.* 11:232–237.

Kraus, MF, Susmaras T, Caughlin BP, et al. 2007. White matter integrity and cognition in chronic traumatic brain injury: a diffusion tensor imaging study. *Brain.* 130(Pt 10):2508–2519.

Kupersmith J, Lew HL, Ommaya AK, et al. 2009. Traumatic brain injury research opportunities: results of Department of Veterans Affairs Consensus Conference (editorial). *J Rehab Res Dev.* 46:VII–XV.

Langlois JA, Rutland-Brown W, Wald MM. 2006. The epidemiology and impact of traumatic brain injury. *J Head Trauma Rehabil.* 21:375–378.

Levin HS, Brown SA, Song JX, et al. 2001. Depression and posttraumatic stress disorder at three months after mild to moderate traumatic brain injury. *J Clin Exp Nueropsychol.* 23:754–769.

Levin HS, Mattis S, Ruff RM, et al. 1987. Neurobehavioral outcome following minor head injury: a three-center study. *J Neurosurg.* 66:234–243.

Lippa SM, Pastorek NJ, Benge JF, Thornton GM. 2010. Postconcussive symptoms after blast and nonblast-related mild traumatic brain injuries in Afghanistan and Iraq War veterans. *J Int Neuropsychol Soc.* 16:856–866.

MacDonald, CL, Johnson, AM, Cooper, D, et al, 2011. Detection of blast-related traumatic brain injury in U.S. military personnel. *NEJM.* 364(22):2091–2100.

MacGregor AJ, Shaffer RA, Dougherty AL, et al. 2010. Prevalence and psychological correlates of traumatic brain injury in Operation Iraqi Freedom. *J Head Trauma Rehabil.* 25:1–8.

McCullagh S, Feinstein A. 2011. Cognitive Changes. In: Silver JM, McAllister TW, Yudofsky SC, editors. *Textbook of Traumatic Brain Injury.* 2nd ed. Arlington, VA: American Psychiatric Publishing, Inc.

Middelboe T, Andersen HS, Birket-Smith M, Friis ML. 1992. Psychiatric sequelae of minor head injury: a prospective follow-up study. *European Psychiatry.* 7:183–189.

Moore DF, Jaffee MS. 2010. Military traumatic brain injury and blast (editorial). *Neuro Rehabilitation.* 26:179–181.

Nelson LA, Yoash-Gantz RE, Pickett TC, Campbell TA. 2009. Relationship between processing speed and executive functioning performance among OEF/OIF veterans: implications for postdeployment rehabilitation. *J Head Trauma Rehabil.* 24:32–40.

Niogi SN, Mukherjee P. 2010. Diffusion tensor imaging of mild traumatic brain injury. *J Head Trauma Rehabil.* 25(4):241–255.

Ohry A, Solomon Z, Rattok J. 1996. Post traumatic stress disorder in traumatic brain injury. *Brain Injury.* 10:687–695.

Owens BD, Kragh JF Jr, Wenke JC, et al. 2008. Combat wounds in operation Iraqi Freedom and Operation Enduring Freedom. *J Trauma.* 64:295–299.

Pietrzak RH, Johnson DC, Goldstein MB, et al. 2009. Posttraumatic stress disorder mediates the relationship between mild traumatic brain injury and health and psychosocial functioning in veterans of Operations Enduring Freedom and Iraqi Freedom. *J Nerv Ment Dis.* 197:748–753.

Pitman RK. 2010. Posttraumatic stress disorder and dementia. What is the origin of the association? *JAMA.*;30;2287–2288.

Ponsford J, Willmott C, Rothwell A., et al. 2000. Factors influencing outcome following mild traumatic brain injury in adults. *J Int Neuropsychol Soc.* 6(5):568–579.

Polusny MA, Kehle SM, Nelson NW, et al. 2011. Longitudinal effects of mild traumatic brain injury and posttraumatic stress disorder comorbidity on postdeployment outcomes in National Guard soldiers deployed to Iraq. *Arch Gen Psychiatry.* 68:79–89.

Rauch SL, Shin LM, Phelps EA. 2006. Neurocircuitry models of posttraumatic stress disorder and extinction: human neuroimaging research—past, present, and future. *Biol Psychiatry.* 60:376–382.

Rogers JM, Read CA. 2007. Psychiatric comorbidity following traumatic brain injury. *Brain Inj.* 21:1321–1333.

Rutgers DR, Toulgoat F, Cazejust J, et al. 2008. White matter abnormalities in mild traumatic brain injury: a diffusion tensor imaging study. *AJNR Am J Neuroradiol.* 29(3):514–519.

Schell TL, Marshall GN. 2008. Survey of individuals previously deployed for OIF/OEF. In: Tanielian T, Jaycox LH, editors. *Invisible Wounds of War: Mental Health and Cognitive Care Needs of America's Returning Veterans.* Santa Monica, CA: RAND Corportion.

Schneiderman AI, Braver ER, Kang HK. 2008. Understanding sequelae of injury mechanisms and mild traumatic brain injury incurred during the conflicts in Iraq and Afghanistan: persistent postconcussive symptoms and posttraumatic stress disorder. *Am J Epidemiol.* 167(12):1446–1452.

Schwab KA, Ivins B, Cramer G, et al. 2007. Screening for traumatic brain injury in troops returning from deployment in Afghanistan and Iraq: initial investigation of the usefulness of a short screening tool for traumatic brain injury. *J Head Trauma Rehabil.* 22:377–389.

Summers CR, Ivins B, Schwab KA. 2009. Traumatic brain injury in the United States: an epidemiologic overview. *Mt Sinai J Med.* 76:105–110.

Tanielian T, Jaycox LH, Schell TL, et al, editors. 2008. *Invisible Wounds of War.* Santa Monica, CA: RAND Corporation.

Teasdale G, Jennett B. 1974. Assessment of coma and impaired consciousness. A practical scale. *Lancet.* 2:81–84.

Terrio H, Brenner LA, Ivins BJ, et al. 2009. Traumatic brain injury screening: preliminary findings in a US Army Brigade Combat Team. *J Head Trauma Rehabil.* 24:14–23.

Terrio HP, Nelson LA, Betthauser LM, et al. 2011. Postdeployment traumatic brain injury screening questions: sensitivity, specificity, and predictive values in returning soldiers. *Rehabil Psychol.* 56:26–31.

Turnbull SJ, Campbell EA, Swann IJ. 2001. Post-traumatic stress disorder symptoms following a head injury: does amnesia for the event influence the development of symptoms? *Brain Inj.* 15(9):775–785.

Vanderploeg RD, Belanger HG, Curtiss G. 2009. Mild traumatic brain injury and posttraumatic stress disorder and their associations with health symptoms. *Arch Phys Med Rehabil.* 90:1084–1093.

Vanderploeg RD, Curtiss G, Luis CA, Salazar AM. 2007. Long-term morbidities following self-reported mild traumatic brain injury. *J Clin Exp Neuropsychol.* 29:585–598.

Van Dyke SA, Axelrod BN, Schutte C. 2010. Test-retest reliability of the Traumatic Brain Injury Screening Instrument. *Mil Med.* 175:947–949.

Van Reekum R, Cohen T, Wong J. 2000. Can traumatic brain injury cause psychiatric disorders? *J Neuropsychiatry Clin Neurosci.* 12:316–327.

Vasterling JJ, Proctor SP, Amoroso P, et al. 2006. Neuropsychological outcomes of army personnel following deployment to the Iraq war. *JAMA.* 296(5):519–529.

Warden D. 2006. Military TBI during the Iraq and Afghanistan wars. *J Head Trauma Rehabil.* 21:398–402.

Warden DL, Ryan LM, Helmick KM, et al. 2005. War neurotrauma: the Defense and Veterans Brain Injury Center (DVBIC) experience at Walter Reed Army Medical Center (WRAMC). *J Neurotrauma.* 22:1178.

Whelan-Goodinson R, Ponsford JL, Johnston L, Grant F. 2009. Predictors of psychiatric disorders following traumatic brain injury. *J Head Trauma Rehabil.* 24:324–332.

Wilde EA, McCauley SR, Hunter JV, et al. 2008. Diffusion tensor imaging of acute mild traumatic brain injury in adolescents. *Neurology.* 70(12):948–955.

Williams WH, Evans JJ, Needham P, Wilson BA. 2002. Neurological, cognitive and attributional predictors of posttraumatic stress symptoms after traumatic brain injury. *J Trauma Stress.* 15:397–400.

Williams WH, Evans JJ, Wilson BA, Needham P. 2002. Brief report: prevalence of post-traumatic stress disorder symptoms after severe traumatic brain injury in a representative community sample. *Brain Inj.* 16:673–679.

Yaffe K, Vittinghoff E, Lindquist K, et al. 2010. Posttraumatic stress disorder and risk of dementia among US veterans. *Arch Gen Psychiatry.* 67:608–613.

Zoroya G. 2006. Pentagon holds brain injury data. *USA Today.*

9

Toward an Improved Understanding of Post-Traumatic Stress Disorder and Chronic Health Conditions

Steven S. Coughlin, Ph.D., and J. Wesson Ashford, M.D., Ph.D.

The chapters included in this book summarize and interpret the sizeable literature on post-traumatic stress disorder (PTSD) and chronic health conditions. They include studies that have contributed to our current understanding of the epidemiology and pathophysiology of PTSD and other psychiatric conditions, substance abuse and dependency, chronic pain, obesity, diabetes, cardiovascular disease, and traumatic brain injury. Related public health and clinical research topics such as PTSD occurring after the diagnosis of myocardial infarction, stroke, HIV/AIDS, or cancer, have also been highlighted. Drawing upon these published studies, the purpose of this concluding chapter is to point to areas where further research is needed and to highlight frameworks and logic models for understanding causal and non-causal relationships between PTSD and chronic health conditions.

FRAMEWORKS FOR UNDERSTANDING CAUSAL RELATIONSHIPS BETWEEN PTSD AND CHRONIC HEALTH CONDITIONS

As highlighted throughout this book, a variety of psychological, neurohormonal, and immunological mechanisms may account for the co-occurrence of PTSD with other medical and psychiatric conditions. In addition to multicausality, the mechanisms that play a key role in the causation of specific comorbidities are likely to vary. General models of possible mechanisms underlying the relationships between PTSD and physical and psychological health have pointed to the hypothalamic-pituitary-adrenal (HPA) axis, heightened noradrenergic function, and immune function, as well as psychological comorbidities such as depression, health risk behaviors, symptom reports, and functional status (Green and Kimerling 2004; Schnurr and Green 2004). Such general models or frameworks have also included genetic influences and history of trauma and stressful life events (Boscarino 2004). The inclusion of psychiatric comorbidity in the models adds important insights. For example, the association of PTSD and borderline personality disorder may be partly accounted for by an exacerbation of the emotion dysregulation that is a core feature of borderline personality disorder (Harned et al. 2010). Persons suffering from PTSD can vacillate between intense emotional reexperiencing and emotional numbing, which could plausibly worsen the disturbances seen in borderline personality disorder and lead to a more complex clinical presentation. Of course, PTSD is unlikely to be the only pathway by which traumatic events lead to adverse health outcomes since trauma can lead to several anxiety and mood disorders and to adverse changes in health risk factors (Schnurr and Green 2004). The co-occurrence of PTSD and traumatic brain injury is partly accounted for by shared exposures (for example, trauma from motor vehicle accidents or combat-related blast injuries).

The sizeable literature on PTSD and alcohol and drug abuse and dependence provides important examples of pathways by which PTSD may lead to substance abuse and dependence, and vice versa. As discussed in Chapter 4, these include the "self-medication" hypothesis which posits that persons with PTSD use psychoactive substances to alleviate their traumatic memories and other painful symptoms, and alcohol or drug abuse is then maintained by negative reinforcement (Chilcoat and Breslau 1998; Kaysen et al. 2007). There has also been increasing interest in developing frameworks for better understanding PTSD occurring in the aftermath of myocardial infarction, cancer, HIV/AIDS, and other potentially life-threatening illnesses, including the effect of PTSD on adherence with treatment recommendations.

Although the published literature indicates that PTSD is likely to be a key pathway through which traumatic exposures lead to important adverse health outcomes including substance abuse and cardiovascular disease (Schnurr and

Green 2004), studies completed to date provide an incomplete understanding of the range of chronic conditions that occur with increased frequency among persons with PTSD and about the direction of causal relationships. Part of the problem is that many studies have been cross-sectional in nature, are based upon selected samples of patients, or have not adequately controlled for potential confounding factors. In addition, there has been wide variation across studies in the approach taken to assess PTSD and co-occurring health conditions (for example, self-reported information versus diagnostic clinical interview). The duration of time elapsed between exposure to trauma and the development of PTSD or comorbidity, and the nature and severity of trauma, has also varied widely across studies.

In considering the causality of associations between PTSD and comorbid conditions, it is helpful to consider the criteria used in epidemiology for evaluating the causality of associations identified in observational research, even though criteria-based methods provide only general guidelines for assessing the causality of associations rather than a strict checklist for identifying a causal relationship (Rothman and Greenland 2005; Ward 2009). These criteria include time order, the strength of the association, consistency, analogy, biological plausibility, coherence, and biological gradient or dose-response curve (Coughlin 2010). Coherence entails the extent to which a hypothesized causal association is compatible with preexisting theory and knowledge (Susser 1991). The directionality of an association between exposure and a disease or other adverse health outcome is often an essential point in deliberations about the causality of an association. Although a suspected causal factor must precede the effect or occur simultaneously with it, there may be feedback loops or mutual causation for some causes and their effects (for example, PTSD leading to substance abuse and substance abuse leading to PTSD). Approaches for clarifying genetic influences in PTSD are also of interest, as discussed in Chapter 1. In epidemiology, directed acyclic graphs have been increasingly used to assess causal relationships such as gene-environment interactions (Coughlin 2010; Geneitti et al. 2011).

NON-CAUSAL EXPLANATIONS FOR PTSD COMORBIDITY

There are also non-causal explanations that may account for some PTSD comorbidity. Clinical populations tend to have more comorbid conditions in general, due to referral patterns and selection biases. Differential diagnosis and patterns of clinical practice may also play a role. As noted in Chapter 3, PTSD has overlapping symptomatology with other psychiatric and medical conditions (for example, panic attacks and major depression). Features of borderline personality disorder may develop in response to PTSD symptoms. The chronic insomnia and nightmares experienced by many persons with PTSD can lead to irritability, anger, and mood changes (Axelrod et al. 2005). Although the co-occurrence of PTSD and alcohol abuse and dependence may be partly due to shared risk factors, there are still likely to be causal relations between PTSD and drug and alcohol dependence. The relationship between PTSD and major depression is of particular interest since both conditions can develop from traumatic exposures and there is some overlap in DSM-IV-TR criteria for PTSD and major depression. Observations that persons with preexisting major depression may be more likely to develop PTSD following a traumatic event lend support to a causal interpretation of the link between major depression and PTSD.

LIFE COURSE APPROACH TO UNDERSTANDING PTSD COMORBIDITY

There has been extensive discussion in the psychiatric and psychological literature of the long-term effects of early adverse life experiences. Studies have shown that adverse experiences during childhood increase risk for subsequent PTSD and that trauma during childhood increases vulnerability for developing PTSD later in life (Bremner et al. 1993; Gunderson and Sabo 1993; Widom 1999; Cabrera et al. 2007). However, relatively few epidemiologic studies have examined the long-term effects of childhood abuse and neglect and other early adverse life experiences on the development of PTSD comorbidities throughout the life course. In the Adverse Childhood Experiences study, adult health maintenance organization patients who reported four or more types of a variety of adverse childhood experiences (sexual, physical, or psychological abuse, exposure to interparental violence, living in a household in which a member was a substance abuser, mentally ill, suicidal, or imprisoned) were more likely to report chronic bronchitis, emphysema, stroke, cancer, and coronary heart disease (Felitti et al. 1998). Longitudinal studies are needed to examine the adverse effects of trauma experienced during childhood and later in life as predictors of medical and psychiatric conditions that co-occur with PTSD. A life-course approach to understanding PTSD and related comorbid conditions also takes into account exposures to extreme stress during key developmental periods (for example, fetal, infancy, childhood, and adolescence) including *in utero* exposures.

ADDITIONAL AREAS WHERE FURTHER RESEARCH IS NEEDED

Much of the published work on PTSD and chronic, comorbid health conditions has focused on four broad areas of investigation: (1) the interrelationships between PTSD and other psychiatric conditions including alcohol and drug abuse and dependence; (2) the occurrence of chronic pain among persons with PTSD; (3) linkages between PTSD and cardiovascular disease; and (4) PTSD and traumatic brain injury. Interpersonal violence, armed conflicts, and heightened risk of terrorism in many parts of the world, accompanied with psychological trauma and mass casualties among civilian and non-civilian populations, as well as concern over large numbers of military personnel and veterans with PTSD and blast-related traumatic brain injury, have added urgency to ongoing and planned epidemiologic and clinical studies of these important health concerns. Another area where there has been a rapid growth of published work on PTSD and chronic, comorbid health conditions is the interrelationships of PTSD and obesity, diabetes, and the metabolic syndrome. The occurrence of PTSD among persons living with cancer and HIV/AIDS are further areas where there has been increasing research.

Despite the burgeoning literature on PTSD and chronic health conditions, many important questions remain to be answered in future studies. Additional research is needed about resilience factors that may protect some individuals from developing PTSD after exposure to extreme stressors. Although resilience factors such as social support, coping style and coping mechanisms, or lack of a prior history of trauma are likely to partly account for why some individuals exposed to traumatic events do not develop PTSD, there are gaps in our current understanding of specific psychological, biological, and genetic factors that may protect against PTSD. A variety of factors may interact to determine the severity and persistence of PTSD, including the cumulative number and salience of traumatic experiences, biological and constitutional factors, and receipt of early medical or psychological intervention (Friedman et al. 2007).

Of particular interest are longitudinal studies that prospectively follow persons exposed to traumatic events and studies of gene-environment interactions and epigenetic influences. In addition, further neurobiological and genetic research is needed to clarify why some trauma survivors recover from PTSD while others do not (Yehuda 2000). There is a need for a better understanding of why some persons suffering from PTSD do not recover over time, even among those who receive high-quality care and evidence-based treatment. As noted in Chapter 3, the co-occurrence of PTSD with major depressive disorder, bipolar illness, or other comorbid psychiatric conditions has been associated with poorer prognosis and higher suicide risk (Campbell et al. 2007).

In areas where there is substantial evidence that PTSD increases risk of adverse health outcomes or leads to greater patient distress, more complex illness, or a poorer prognosis (for example, PTSD and substance abuse and dependence), prospective studies are needed to better understand how treatment for comorbid conditions affects recovery from PTSD, and vice versa. Many observational studies of PTSD comorbidity have been cross-sectional in nature and have not examined whether research participants received treatment for PTSD or comorbid psychiatric conditions over time. Although the effectiveness of dual-diagnosis treatment programs has been examined in evaluative studies, and additional trials of dual-diagnosis treatment programs are needed (Gulliver and Steffen 2010), randomized controlled trials have sometimes been criticized for failing to predict real-world outcomes (Sullivan and Goldmann 2011). Clinical trials tend to provide information about the efficacy of interventions under ideal conditions and sometimes exclude patients with complex or overlapping medical or psychiatric conditions. In contrast, comparative effectiveness research focuses on the effectiveness of interventions under average conditions in diverse populations and clinical practice settings (Rich 2009). Both randomized clinical trials and nonrandomized, observational studies provide important information (Dreyer et al. 2010). There is a need for patient-centered comparative effectiveness research of dual-diagnosis treatment programs and other innovative therapies for PTSD, including prospective studies that utilize state-of-the art data-mining techniques applied to administrative databases and electronic medical records. Databases that include recorded measures of functional status, quality of life, and pharmacological and psychological treatments would be espicially helpful for this purpose (Sullivan and Goldmann 2011). Patient-centered comparative effectiveness research is likely to be helpful for identifying which PTSD patients and other survivors of traumatic exposures are most likely to benefit from innovative treatments and to accelerative innovation into clinical practice (Slutsky and Clancy 2010).

Areas where further efforts are needed include longitudinal studies of neurological conditions and PTSD. As discussed in Chapter 8, major advances have been made in applying structural and functional neuroimaging techniques to gaining a better understanding of the physiological processes that are altered in PTSD. However, few neuroimaging studies have looked at changes in brain structure or function over long periods of time, even though studies to date highlight the neuroplasticity of brain structures such as the hypothalamus. Neuroimaging studies of veteran populations do not take into account brain structure and function prior to or during military deployment. The imaging is often done long after, sometimes several years following the period during which combat-related exposures and other extreme stressors are most likely to have occurred. Preliminary evidence of associations between PTSD and dementia (Yaffe et al. 2010; Pitman 2010) and stroke (Coughlin 2011) underscore the need for longitudinal studies of neurological outcomes among persons with and without PTSD, including studies that can help clarify pathophysiological mechanisms.

Comorbidity between PTSD and asthma, chronic bronchitis, or emphysema is another area ripe for further research. Studies have shown that psychological stress can exacerbate childhood asthma by altering the magnitude of airway inflammatory responses to irritants, allergens, and infections (Chen and Miller 2007). The biological pathways that account for how stress amplifies immune responses to asthma triggers include the HPA axis and the autonomic nervous system (Chen and Miller 2007; Priftis and Chrousos 2009). Of course, many populations exposed to psychological trauma are also potentially exposed to environmental dusts and irritants. Examples of the latter include children in Manhattan following the September 11, 2001, terrorist attacks (Szema et al. 2009), persons in New Orleans in the wake of Hurricane Katrina (Rabito et al. 2007), U.S. soldiers serving in Iraq and Afghanistan (Szema et al. 2010), and Australian firefighters suffering from PTSD (McFarlane et al. 1994).

Another area of active research is the relationship between PTSD and autoimmune diseases such as rheumatoid arthritis. The joint inflammation and destruction that is seen in rheumatoid arthritis is partly due to cell-mediated immune responses and the production of autoantibodies (Janeway and Travers 1994). Psychological trauma and stressful events are likely associated with symptom flare-ups or other changes in disease activity (Dougall and Baum 2004).

The relationship between PTSD and women's health concerns is also important to address in future research. There is an ongoing need to better understand physiological pathways that contribute to gender disparities in PTSD and other trauma-related health conditions. As noted in Chapter 3, observations from epidemiologic studies indicate that gender may moderate associations between traumatic exposures and PTSD. Studies of immune function in persons with PTSD (for example, secretion of proinflammatory cytokines such as interleukin-6) may help to clarify the biological under-pinnings of gender disparities in trauma-related adverse health conditions such as autoimmune conditions that are more prevalent among women (Kimerling, 2004; Gill et al. 2005).

REFERENCES

Boscarino JA. 2004. Posttraumatic stress disorder and physical illness. Results from clinical and epidemiologic studies. *Ann NY Acad Sci.* 1032:141–153.

Bremner JD, Southwick SM, Johnson DR, et al. 1993. Childhood physical abuse and combat-related posttraumatic stress disorder in Vietnam veterans. *Am J Psychiatry.* 150:235–239.

Cabrera OA, Hoge CW, Bliese PD, et al. 2007. Childhood adversity and combat as predictors of depression and post-traumatic stress in deployed troops. *Am J Prev Med.* 33:77–82.

Campbell DG, Felker ML, Liu CF, et al. 2007. Prevalence of depression-PTSD comorbidity: implications for clinical practice guidelines and primary care-based interventions. *J Gen Int Med.* 22:711–718.

Chen E, Miller GE. 2007. Stress and inflammation in exacerbations of asthma. *Brain Behav Immun.* 21:993–9.

Chilcoat HD, Breslau N. 1998. Posttraumatic stress disorder and drug disorders: testing causal pathways. *Arch Gen Psychiatry.* 55:913–917.

Coughlin SS. 2011. Post-traumatic stress disorder and cardiovascular disease. *The Open Cardiovascular Medicine Journal.* 5.

Coughlin SS. 2010. Causal Inference and Scientific Paradigms in Epidemiology. Bentham Scientific Publishing.

Dougall AL, Baum A. 2004. Psychoneuroimmunology and trauma. In: Schnurr PP, Green BL, editors. *Trauma and Health: Physical Health Consequences of Exposure to Extreme Stress.* Washington DC: American Psychological Association: 129–155.

Dreyer NA, Tunis SR, Berger M, et al. 2010. Why observational studies should be among the tools used in comparative effectiveness research. *Health Aff (Millwood).* 29:1818–1825.

Felitti VJ, Anda RF, Nordenberg D, et al. 1998. Relationship of childhood abuse and household dysfunction to many of the leading causes of death in adults: The Adverse Childhood Experiences (ACE) study. *Am J Prev Med.* 14:245–258.

Friedman MJ, Keane TM, Resnick PA, editors. 2007. *Handbook of PTSD: Science and Practice.* New York: Guilford Press.

Geneletti SG, Gallo V, Porta M, et al. 2011. Assessing causal relationships in genomics: from Bradford-Hill criteria to complex gene-environment interactions and directed acyclic graphs. *Emerg Themes Epidemiol.* 8:5

Gill JM, Szanton SL, Page GG. 2005. biological underpinnings of health alterations in women with PTSD: a sex disparity. *Biol Res Nurs.* 7:44–54.

Green BL, Kimerling R. 2004. Trauma, posttraumatic stress disorder, and health status. In: Schnurr PP, Green BL, editors. 2004. *Trauma and Health: Physical Consequences of Exposure to Extreme Stress.* Washington, DC: American Psychological Association. 13–42.

Gulliver SB, Steffen LE. 2010. Towards integrated treatments for PTSD and substance use disorders. *PTSD Research Quarterly.* 21:1–7.

Gunderson JG, Sabo AN. 1993. The phenomenological and conceptual interface between borderline personality disorder and PTSD. *Am J Psychiatry.* 150:19–27.

Harned MS, Rizvi SL, Linehan MM. 2010. Impact of co-occurring posttraumatic stress disorder on suicidal women with borderline personality disorder. *Am J Psychiatry.* 167:1210–1217.

Janeway CA, Jr, Travers P. 1994. *Immunobiology: The Immune System in Health and Disease.* New York: Garland Publishing.

Kaysen D, Simpson T, Dillworth T, et al. 2006. Alcohol problems and posttraumatic stress disorder in female crime victims. *J Trauma Stress.* 19:399–403.

Kaysen D, Dillworth TM, Simpson T, et al. 2007. Domestic violence and alcohol use: trauma-related symptoms and motives for drinking. *Addict Behav.* 32:1272–1283.

Kimerling R. 2004. An investigation of sex differences in non-psychiatric morbidity associated with posttraumatic stress disorder. *J Am Med Womens Assoc.* 59:43–47.

Pitman RK. 2010. Posttraumatic stress disorder and dementia. What is the origin of the association? 303:2287–2288.

Prifitis KN, Chrousos GP. 2009. Neuroimmunomodulation in asthma: focus on the hypothalamic-pituitary-adrenal axis. *Neuroimmunomodulation.* 16:263–264.

Rabito FA, Iqbal S, Kiernan MP, et al. 2008. Children's Respiratory Health and Mold Levels in New Orleans Post-Katrina: A preliminary look. *J Asthma Clin Immunol.* 121:622–625.

Rich EC. 2009. The policy debate over public investment in comparative effectiveness research. *J Gen Intern Med.* 24:752–757.

Rothman KJ, Greenland S. 2005. Causation and causal inference in epidemiology. *Am J Public Health.* 95:S144–S150.

Schnurr PP, Green BL. 2004. Understanding relationships among trauma, post-traumatic stress disorder, and health outcomes. *Advances.* 20:18–29.

Slutsky JR, Clancy CM. 2010. Patient-centered comparative effectiveness research. Essential for high-quality care. *Arch Int Med.* 170:403–404.

Sullivan P, Goldmann D. 2011. The promise of comparative effectiveness research. *JAMA.* 305:400–401.

Susser M. 1991. What is a cause and how do we know one? A grammar for pragmatic epidemiology. *Am J Epidemiol.* 133:635–648.

Szema AM, Savary KW, Ying BL, Lai K. 2009. Post 9/11: high asthma rates among children in Chinatown, New York. *Allergy Asthma Proc.* 30:605–611.

Szema AM, Peters MC, Weissinger KM, et al. 2010. New-onset asthma among soldiers serving in Iraq and Afghanistan. *Allergy Asthma Proc.* 31:67–71.

Ward A. 2009. Causal criteria and the problem of complex causation. *Med Health Care Philos.* 12:333–343.

Widom CS. 1999. Posttraumatic stress disorder in abused and neglected children grown up. *Am J Psychiatry.* 156:1223–1229.

Yaffe K, Vittinghoff E, Lindquist K, et al. 2010. Post-traumatic stress disorder and risk of dementia among U.S. veterans. *Arch Gen Psychiatry.* 67:608–613.

Yehuda R. Biology of posttraumatic stress disorder. 2000. *J Clin Psychiatry.* 61(Suppl 7):14–21.

Subject Index

2